SpringerBriefs in Public Health present concise summaries of cutting-edge research and practical applications from across the entire field of public health, with contributions from medicine, bioethics, health economics, public policy, biostatistics, and sociology.

The focus of the series is to highlight current topics in public health of interest to a global audience, including health care policy; social determinants of health; health issues in developing countries; new research methods; chronic and infectious disease epidemics; and innovative health interventions.

Featuring compact volumes of 50 to 125 pages, the series covers a range of content from professional to academic. Possible volumes in the series may consist of timely reports of state-of-the art analytical techniques, reports from the field, snapshots of hot and/or emerging topics, literature reviews, and in-depth case studies. Both solicited and unsolicited manuscripts are considered for publication in this series.

Briefs are published as part of Springer's eBook collection, with millions of users worldwide. In addition, Briefs are available for individual print and electronic purchase.

Briefs are characterized by fast, global electronic dissemination, standard publishing contracts, easy-to-use manuscript preparation and formatting guidelines, and expedited production schedules. We aim for publication 8–12 weeks after acceptance.

Amos Laar

# Balancing the Socio-political and Medico-ethical Dimensions of HIV

A Social Public Health Approach

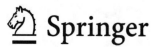 Springer

Amos Laar
Department of Population, Family, and Reproductive Health, School of Public Health,
College of Health Sciences
University of Ghana
Accra, Ghana

ISSN 2192-3698          ISSN 2192-3701    (electronic)
SpringerBriefs in Public Health
ISBN 978-3-031-09190-2          ISBN 978-3-031-09191-9   (eBook)
https://doi.org/10.1007/978-3-031-09191-9

This Springer imprint is published by the registered company Springer Nature Switzerland AG
The registered company address is: Gewerbestrasse 11, 6330 Cham, Switzerland

*I dedicate this book to my family. Ava Chloe, Elia Zoey, Hans Lael, Amos Ethan, and Matilda Laar, you did without me for far too long because of this, and related assignments.*

*To my extended family – although too numerous to name, I must mention Dr. Alexander Laar (my big brother) and my mom (Afia Konduuk Laar) for their unfailing support. My Dad (Duut Laar) and "Uncle Paul" (Mr. Paul Moferi) – both of blessed memory.*

*To my professional family including Dr. W. B. Owusu, Emerita Professor Isabella A. Quakyi, and Emeritus Professor Ebenezer E. Laing (of blessed memory) for initiating me to different aspects of academic life.*

*To the hundreds, thousands, and millions of HIV-infected and affected persons in Ghana and across the globe, I dedicate this book to you.*

# Foreword

Dr. Amos Laar's *Balancing the Socio-political and Medico-ethical Dimensions of HIV: A Social Public Health Approach* offers a powerful vision for reform of the HIV/AIDS response in Ghana and similar settings in the Global South. This vision is grounded in Dr. Laar's strong conviction about the foundational importance of social justice to public health, and manifests his ardent determination to promote well-being in the complex contexts in which the challenges of public health arise. His analysis in this volume demonstrates that a morally appropriate public health response to HIV/AIDS must move beyond a predominant focus on medical intervention, to acknowledge and address the social, cultural, and political context that substantially shapes the course of a pandemic and deeply affects the success of public health measures to protect the population's health.

The analysis requires a broad, interdisciplinary lens to incorporate consideration of this complex context. Thus, Dr. Laar carefully articulates frameworks from ethics, public health, public policy, and social science that are critical to understanding the complex challenges of HIV/AIDS response in the Global South. He further draws from his broad public health expertise to highlight successes in areas other than HIV/AIDS response, to allow for cross-pollination of ideas. For example, given his extensive experience concerning public health nutrition, he considers what lessons for ethical and sustainable HIV/AIDS response might be drawn from extant advocacy and scholar activism movements in public health nutrition. He also situates discussion of the current HIV/AIDS response in its historic context. Doing so fosters understanding of how the past has shaped the current response, and allows the reader to appreciate influences on public health that may be invisible if we confined our attention to the present. It also provides important context for understanding HIV/AIDS denialism and conspiracy theories, to promote the ability to address these challenges.

Moreover, Dr. Laar recognizes that, to evaluate the moral appropriateness of HIV/AIDS response measures, the analysis should not only consider quantitative data about matters such as case rates and access to therapies but must also heed the lived experiences of people confronting the realities of HIV/AIDS in Africa. He includes these voices with sensitivity and respect, as a critical feature of the analysis. He wisely appreciates that we can learn a great deal from the narratives of both individuals who are HIV-positive and those who are HIV-negative. They all contain insights gleaned from witnessing the HIV/AIDS pandemic, confronting its risks, and navigating the social, cultural, and political context of the pandemic and response to it.

This thoughtful engagement with community members also reflects Dr. Laar's commitment to respect the rights of individuals – a commitment that is central to public health's code of ethics, but which is all too often overlooked in the practice of public health. The volume shines a light on structural violence – the systemic inequities that can undermine the ability of individuals or populations to meet their basic needs, let alone realize their right to their highest attainable level of health. In particular, the analysis demonstrates how rights-limiting policies – such as Ghana's penalties for the behaviors of sex workers and men who have sex with men – undercut HIV/AIDS response by increasing risk, not only in these populations but also in the population at large.

Thus, Dr. Laar uses this volume to speak truth to power, to advocate for a morally appropriate response to HIV/AIDS in the Global South. He demonstrates that the discussion must include far more than the typical considerations of the effectiveness of preventive measures and therapies and the population's access – or lack thereof – to these resources. It must consider social and cultural norms and realities, rights and power, and the ways that all of these forces intersect with public health. The relative scarcity of preventive and treatment resources does hamper HIV/AIDS response in this context, but Dr. Laar conclusively demonstrates that promoting an effective and equitable response requires a paradigm shift to social public health.

The volume offers a compelling read for a wide audience, including public health leaders and practitioners, policy makers, social science scholars, ethicists, and the media. It provides a knowledgeable, well-grounded, and morally sensitive examination of the possibilities – and limits – of advocacy movements in addressing the urgent challenges of the HIV/AIDS pandemic in Ghana and the Global South more generally. I hope that it inspires a diverse array of stakeholders to work for health justice.

Minneapolis, MN, USA                                                            Debra DeBruin
November 2021

# Preface

"All die be die" is a provocative political statement in Ghana. But it is also a statement public health advocates and vulnerable, socially excluded persons have used to convey the obstacles to change in the face of HIV infection in Ghana. The statement is emblematic of the challenges that individuals infected with, or affected by HIV, deal with, as they strive to make meaning of life. Interventions to address HIV and AIDS must recognize that the social, economic, or political influencers of people's behavior and choices, in some instances, trump medical rationalizations. Some people are going to die anyway, and it may not matter much what they die from. "Dying from AIDS through sex work is not different from dying from any other disease, or from hunger" unpacks a renowned Ghanaian Professor (Kofi Awusabo-Asare). As national policy professionals, programmers, and public health professionals design and implement interventions to respond to AIDS, these ought to be paid heed to.

Indeed, responding to public health challenges whether at the global or local levels can give rise to an array of tensions. To assure sustainable public health, these tensions need to be meaningfully and sufficiently balanced. Using empirical evidence and lived experiences from the Global South, this book enunciates the many dimensions of national-level responses to HIV or AIDS. Calling out glaring neglects, the book offers a rare critical perspective of public health response to AIDS in Ghana. Invoking the philosophy of social public health, the book makes a case for the destabilization of the naturalness with which national AIDS responses ignore its (AIDS') socio-political and medico-ethical dimensions. Although presented as a case study, this critical perspective is not unique to Ghana's response to AIDS; it may well serve as an illustrative voice for similarly situated settings globally. Second, although the book draws principally from empirical evidence and lived experiences relating to AIDS, it is deliberately loaded with relevant public health concepts, and philosophies, and thus articulates insights beyond a single disease condition. As such, the book makes a compelling read for a broad spectrum of scholars, professionals, and students interested in public health, public policy, social sciences, bioethics, medical anthropologists, sociologists, global health scholars, and medicine. Public health economists, lay politicians, and civil society organizations advocating for health equity will also find the book useful. Written at a time when public health actors are repositioning themselves to be competent users of not only pharmacologic vaccines but also social vaccines, the book is timely.

Accra, Ghana                                                                      Amos Laar

# Acknowledgments

This book could not have been written without the support and contributions of many. The funding from the Ghana National AIDS Control Programme (NACP) – toward the implementation of my BSc project – in 2003 played a pivotal role in this journey. This gesture from the NACP piqued my interest in HIV research, and would keep me there for over a decade – exploring the socio-cultural, socio-ethical, and medico-ethical dimensions of HIV. To which I owe monumental gratitude to Dr. Kwaku Yeboah, erstwhile program manager, NACP.

The contributions from my professional family including Dr. W. B. Owusu, Emerita Professor Isabella A. Quakyi, and Emeritus Professor Ebenezer E. Laing (of blessed memory), all of the University of Ghana, Emerita Professor Amy Tsui (Johns Hopkins Bloomberg School of Public Health), and Dr. Alexander Laar to my academic life cannot go unacknowledged.

This book benefits from the rich experiences from and encounters with members of the School of Public Health TALIF HIV Initiative, as well as the HIV360 Research and Practice Consortium. I am grateful to the various entities that provided financial support toward my HIV work. These include – in no particular order – the HIV Research Trust Fund of the United Kingdom, the Ghana AIDS Commission, the University of Ghana, Gates Institute at Johns Hopkins University, Measure Evaluation, the Canadian International Development Research Center (IDRC), the World Bank's TALIF initiative. The United Nations World Food Programme and the Ghana AIDS Commission, on two occasions, offered me the opportunity to lead the assessment of a nationwide food security and vulnerability assessment of Ghanaian HIV-affected households. Serving as a consultant to the Global Fund, to the UNAIDS, and several others have impacted my appreciation of the various dimensions of HIV.

The University of Minnesota, Center for Bioethics – my alma mater – offered me a slot to speak at their prestigious "Ethics Ground Rounds Series." Titled "Social Public Health and Ghana National Response to HIV," this book metamorphosed from the talk.

Dr. Ireneous Soyiri provided proofreading services and critical editorial support. I would also like to express my gratitude to the early career researchers and associates of my lab – Mr. Silver Nanema, Mr. Gideon Amevinya, Ms. Akosua Pokua Adjei, Ms. Akua Tandoh, Dr. Phyllis Ohene-Agyei, Mr. Emmanuel Hammond, Ms. Justine Koomson, and Lily Egyir for their literature, formatting, and helpful editorial support.

Indebtedness to my family: Ava Chloe, Elia Zoey, Hans Lael, Amos Ethan, and Matilda Laar.

# Contents

# List of Figures

# List of Tables

# About the Author

**Amos Laar, PhD** obtained his BSc (in nutrition and biochemistry), MPH, and PhD (in public health) from the University of Ghana, and MA (in bioethics) from the University of Minnesota, USA. He is a bioethicist and a tenure-track academic in the School of Public Health, University of Ghana, Accra, Ghana. His earlier work makes significant contribution to public health scholarship on women's reproductive health, particularly the socio-cultural, socio-ethical, and medico-ethical dimensions of HIV. Currently his research and professional practice straddle three distinct, yet related areas of public health: bioethics, public health nutrition, and social public health. Through these, his scholarship contributes to a deeper understanding of how physical environments, social environments, and structural forces affect realization of health. He has authored over 90 scholarly works on the above topics. He is a mentor – having supervised over 70 graduate and undergraduate theses from universities in Africa (University of Ghana, University of South Africa), Asia (Nagasaki University of Japan), Europe (University of Sheffield, UK), and North America (University of South Carolina, USA).

# Abbreviations

| | |
|---|---|
| ABC | Abstinence, be faithful and use a condom |
| ACT UP | AIDS Coalition to Unleash Power |
| AFASS | Acceptability, Feasibility, Affordability, Sustainability and Safety |
| AIDS | Acquired Immunodeficiency Syndrome |
| ART | Antiretroviral Therapy |
| ARV | Associated Retrovirus |
| ARVs | Antiretrovirals |
| AZT | Azidothymidine |
| CDC | Centers for Disease Control and Prevention |
| CHRAJ | Commission on Human Rights and Administrative Justice |
| COVID-19 | Coronavirus disease |
| CRS | Catholic Relief Services |
| CSDH | Commission on Social Determinants of Health |
| DANIDA | Danish International Development Agency |
| ddC | Zalcitabine |
| ddI | didanosine/2′,3′-dideoxyinosine |
| DICs | Drop-in Centers |
| ELISA | Enzyme-Linked Immunosorbent Assay |
| eMTCT | elimination of Mother to Child Transmission |
| FDA | Food and Drug Administration |
| FSW | Female Sex Workers |
| GAC | Ghana AIDS Commission |
| GDHS | Ghana Demographic and Health Survey |
| GDP | Gross Domestic Product |
| GRID | Gay-Related Immune Deficiency |
| HAART | Highly Active Anti-Retroviral Therapy |
| HIV | Human Immunodeficiency Virus |
| HTC | HIV Testing and Counselling |
| HTLV-III | Human T-lymphotrophic Virus III |
| HTS | HIV Testing Services |
| ICCPR | International Covenant on Civil and Political Rights |

| | |
|---|---|
| ICESCR | International Covenant on Economic, Social and Cultural Rights |
| IOM | Institute of Medicine |
| iPrEx trial | Pre-exposure trial |
| IRIS | Immune Reconstitution Syndrome |
| KPs | Key Populations |
| LAV | Lymphadenopathy Associated Virus |
| LGBTQIAP | Lesbian, Gay, Bisexual, Transgender, Queer and Questioning, Intersex, Asexual and Pansexual |
| LMIC | Lower Middle-Income Country |
| MARPs | Most-at-Risk Populations |
| MDGs | Millennium Development Goals |
| MOH | Ministry of Health |
| MSM | Men who have Sex with Men |
| MTCT | Mother-to-Child Transmission |
| NAC | National Advisory Commission |
| NACP | National AIDS/STI Control Programme |
| NCDs | Non-Communicable Diseases |
| NGOs | Non-Governmental Organizations |
| NIH | National Institutes of Health |
| NSF | National Strategic Framework |
| NSP | National Strategic Plans |
| PCP | Pneumocystis Carinii Pneumonia |
| PEPFAR | President's Emergency Fund for AIDS Relief |
| PHC | Primary Healthcare |
| PHEIC | Public Health Emergency of International Concern |
| PLWH/PLHIV | Persons Living with HIV |
| PMTCT | Prevention of Mother-to-Child Transmission |
| PrEP | Pre-exposure prophylaxis |
| PWIDs | Persons Who Inject Drugs |
| SDGs | Sustainable Development Goals |
| SSA | Sub-Saharan Africa |
| STDs | Sexually Transmitted Diseases |
| STI | Sexually Transmitted Infection |
| SWs | Sex Workers |
| TasP | Treatment as Prevention |
| TB | Tuberculosis |
| TFM | Transitional Funding Mechanism |
| U = U | Undetectable = Untransmittable |
| UDHR | Universal Declaration of Human Rights |
| UHC | Universal Health Coverage |
| UN | United Nations |
| UNESCO | United Nations Educational, Scientific and Cultural Organization |
| UNGASS | United Nations General Assembly Special Session |
| UNAIDS | Joint United Nations Programme on HIV/AIDS |
| USAID | United States Agency for International Development |

| VCT | Voluntary Counseling and Testing |
| VMMC | Voluntary Male Medical Circumcision |
| WFP | World Food Programme |
| WHO | World Health Organization |

# Chapter 1
# The Practice of Public Health

## 1.1 Introduction

Health and therefore public health are concepts with far-reaching medical but also socio-political implications. Over the years, efforts to find a sociologically, politically, spiritually, and culturally sound cleavage between health as defined and health as experienced in different settings have been met with real challenges [1]. Scholars have attributed this lack of consensus to the complex, interdisciplinary, biopsychosocial, socio-political, and spirito-cultural dimensions of health. While there have been several attempts to rebalance the dominant biomedically weighted conceptions of health, other concepts such as social public health have had limited use in health literature. Laar et al.'s [1] review of the concepts of health and their nuanced analysis of how both medical and indigenous African perspectives of health are important in global public health is relevant here. The following three paragraphs derive principally from this earlier work by Laar et al. [1].

Historically, good health, irrespective of setting, geography, or culture, had been viewed as a supernatural gift from the gods, and disease, a punishment from the same source. As a result, prayers and sacrifices were/are often offered to the gods for "good health," in the quest for healing, and to spare individuals and populations of the misfortune of "bad health" [2]. Medical and philosophical texts from the sixth to fourth centuries BC confirm that the ancient Greeks were the first to break away from supernatural, non-biologic conceptions of health and disease [3]. Humanity's understanding of health has since undergone significant transformations. Following the foundational work of Hippocrates, Galen (130 AD–201 AD) further developed the theory and practice and carried Greco-Roman medicine to its zenith [4]. The miasma theory of health, the idea that bad air "miasma" was the cause of disease, became popular from the first century BC to the middle ages (1880) [5, 6]. Then came the spontaneous generation theory, which suggested that living things arose from non-living matter [7]. Undoubtedly, the work of Francesco Redi, Louis Pasteur, and Robert Koch clarified the existence of germs; thus the germ theory era began [8, 9]. From holistic wellness to germ theory, the evolution of health has been significant. The definition of health has changed from its supernatural and metaphysical foundations to a broader but idealistic conceptualization as captured by the World Health Organization (WHO). Contained in the Constitution of the WHO, health is defined as a state of complete physical, mental, and social well-being and not merely the absence of disease or infirmity [10]. An important definitional perspective emphasizes the point that "social and personal resources as well as physical capabilities" are all important elements for the health of the community. Alongside the WHO's, several definitions of health exist. None has so far been able to give a universally acceptable, yet culturally sensitive, appeal to all [11]. I agree. Many concepts of health, more often than not, fail to accommodate the indigenous knowledge (especially of the African), which are usually deeply rooted in the socio-cultural and spiritual realms. Calls for a renewed debate on how to integrate all concepts into a more contextualized and acceptable global representations of health [1].

## 1.2   Indigenous African Concepts of Health

Although indigenous or aboriginal approaches to health are often rooted in a holistic conception of well-being involving a healthy balance of four elements or aspects of wellness, physical, emotional, mental, and spiritual [12], such conceptions are often portrayed from a deficit-based lens. Several efforts across the globe exist to valorize indigenous conceptions of health. A recent review by Thiessen et al. aimed to systematically map the literature on perspectives, concepts, and constructs of wellness and well-being in indigenous communities across Canada [13]. As noted earlier, Laar et al. advocated for a debate on the contribution of indigenous African conceptions of health in the global health literature and practice. A manifesto by Bacchetta et al. called for the valorization of wild edible plants used by indigenous populations for food and health [14]. As with other indigenous communities across the globe, many indigenous African conceptions of health and illness are deeply rooted in the spiritual realm [15], with the belief that what is seen in the physical realm is inherently controlled by the spiritual [15]. In Africa, people tend to see health as the ability to maintain specific functions, i.e., working and fulfilling societal roles, contributing to the home and fulfilling familial roles, and/or worshipping and contributing to the community's religious or spiritual wellness [16]. Omonzejele for instance had noted that, the traditional African concepts of health go beyond the "living," pivoting around family members, community, and ancestors in the other world [17]. This integrated view of health is based on the African view of reality [17] where intra-relationships are just as important as interrelationships.

It's believed that African indigenous concepts of health and illness do not disregard western medicine. Oti-Boadi, however, qualifies that ill health is ill health but not all ill health can be cured by physical or psychological/social therapies (of western tradition); other more powerful means are needed for special illnesses [18].

While the specific source of power is debatable, that which is common knowledge is the procreation of this power or belief systems. It's transmitted from generation to generation in a familial fashion [15]. The authors characterize such generational transfer of beliefs and its influence on thinking and behavior, including the conceptualization of health, well-being, and illness through this dogma, as "behavior genetics" [15]. Even for some elite Africans who may be health literate (based on the western conception of health), illness and health typically operate within a duality, with a spiritual current running alongside the biopsychosocial "causes." It is of paramount importance that these varied conceptions of health or ill health are recognized in public health and public health practice.

## 1.3 Public Health Practice

As a professional practice, public health is generally conceptualized as the science (but also art) of preventing disease, prolonging life, and promoting health (social, physical, or mental health) of individuals and of their communities. So conceptualized, public health involves the application of many different disciplines – from biology, public policy, statistics, engineering, medicine, public health nursing, nutrition, health education, sociology, anthropology, and business just to name a few. Public health interfaces with and engages stakeholders from every discipline – to accomplish its goals and to serve its mission. These are delivered through several services – the so-called essential public health services. Currently ten in number, these services according to [19] seek to:

- Monitor health status to identify community health problems.
- Diagnose and investigate health problems and health hazards in the community.
- Inform, educate, and empower people about health issues.
- Mobilize community partnerships to identify and solve health problems.
- Develop policies and plans that support individual and community health efforts.
- Enforce laws and regulations that protect health and ensure safety.
- Link people to needed personal health services, and assure the provision of healthcare when otherwise unavailable.
- Assure a competent public and personal healthcare work force.
- Evaluate effectiveness, accessibility, and quality of personal and population-based health services.
- Provide research for new insights and innovative solutions to health problems.

These services recognize the multi-layered determinants of public health (including social, legal, as well as commercial). For instance, the social environment determines health risks (low income and education levels, overcrowding, and personal safety). Other social factors related to the use of health and medical services, such as travel distance, the number of providers, and even the availability of day-care services, also influence health. With so many elements, actors, stakeholders, and sectors affecting health, no one field can claim public health practice, and there is no need to. The purpose of public health practice is to assure health. It does not matter where it is "housed." Health is assured through purposeful actions that prevent, manage, treat, control, eliminate, and if feasible eradicate diseases or health problems. At this point it's apropos to discriminate among these and reiterate the hierarchy of these public health efforts in dealing with infectious diseases (now includes non-infectious diseases or public health problems in general) [20, 21]:

- *Prevention*: the specific, population-based, and individual-based interventions for preventing the occurrence of a disease/health problem (primary prevention), early detection (secondary prevention), and treatment to prevent complications (tertiary prevention. As used here, preventative treatment can include patient education, lifestyle modification, and drugs.
- *Control*: reduction of disease incidence, prevalence, morbidity, or mortality to a locally acceptable level as a result of deliberate efforts. Continued intervention measures are required to maintain the reduction. An example is diarrheal diseases.
- *Elimination*: reduction to zero of the incidence of a specified infection/disease in a defined geographical area as a result of deliberate efforts. Like control, continued intervention measures are required, e.g., measles and poliomyelitis.
- *Eradication*: permanent reduction to zero of the worldwide incidence of infection caused by a specific agent as a result of deliberate efforts; intervention measures are no longer needed. Example is smallpox.
- *Extinction*: the specific infectious agent no longer exists in nature or in the laboratory. Example: none.

I highlight in the following sections, a select age-old public health practices that have endured.

## 1.4   Surveillance

Disease, epidemiologic, or public health surveillance is defined as the ongoing systematic collection, analysis, and interpretation of data and the timely dissemination of these data to those responsible for preventing and controlling disease and injury [22]. Declich and Carter [23] present the historical origins, methods, and evaluation of public health surveillance. They bemoan that although the approach has grown into a complete discipline, within public health, its growth has not been accompanied by parallel growth in the literature about its principles and methods (Desclich and Cater, 1994). In the public health literature and practice, aside from surveillance, testing, screening, and case finding are relevant tools and are commonly used. Testing is usually described as the application of a measurement to select individuals or a case (e.g., animals) for the purpose of identifying a disease or medical condition. The selection of the individuals or animals might be motivated by clinical reason or risk factors that suggest the presence of the condition. Commonly instituted for the purpose of case finding, screening generally refers to the application of a test to all individuals in a defined population. Case finding means identifying a previously unknown or unrecognized condition in apparently healthy or asymptomatic persons   and   offering   pre-symptomatic   "treatment"   (or   other   appropriate interventions) to those so identified. Screening is also sometimes done for surveillance purposes: to monitor the incidence or prevalence of a disease in a defined population over time or to compare the incidence or prevalence among different populations. Other public health practices used to protect the public by preventing exposure to people who have or may have a contagious disease are solation and quarantine. Isolation is done usually to separate sick people with a contagious disease from people who are not sick. Quarantine separates and restricts the movement of people who have been or may have been exposed to a contagious disease. These people may have been exposed to a disease and do not know it, or they may have the disease but do not show symptoms. Of note, isolation is technically and ethically sensible even if a person exposed and infected does not know or does not have symptoms. In implementing these practices, governments may invoke their constitutional powers – sometimes referred to as "the police power" of the state or pandemic mandates. The "police power" is the capacity of the state to regulate behavior and enforce order within their territory for the betterment of the health and to promote the public health safety, morals, and general welfare of their inhabitants [24–26].

## 1.5   Public Health Research Versus Public Health Practice

As embodied in the definition of public health, the skills and competencies necessary for public health practice are both individual and collective. The practice entails policy formulation, program implementation, or service delivery but also investigations. Often scientific and clinical activities are sometimes undertaken by public health agencies. This is sometimes misconstrued as medical research. It is not! Please see illustrations in Fig. 1.1. Otto et al. [27] offer a framework for appreciating

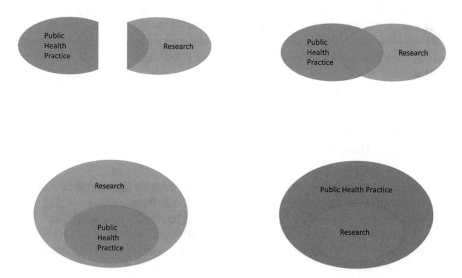

**Fig. 1.1**  Delineating research from public health practice. (Source: Author's construction)

and discriminating between public health practice activities [28] and public health research activities and those that are common to both of them. Since the early 1980s, bioethics scholarship and research ethics guidelines have identified concerns about the boundaries between research and standard clinical care [29, 30]. In 1982, Appelbaum and colleagues documented failure by research participants to appreciate the difference between research and treatment (clinical practice); they coined the term "therapeutic misconception" for the phenomenon [30]. Therapeutic misconception connotes misunderstanding of the research purpose or conflation of research with clinical practice or public health practice. Others have distinguished therapeutic misestimation and therapeutic optimism from therapeutic misconception [31]. Therapeutic misestimation means misestimating the chance of benefit or risk associated with a research practice (i.e., overestimating or underestimating risk). Therapeutic optimism on the other hand is present when a research participant expresses the view that he/she will benefit from participation in a trial that offers its participants little or no prospect for direct medical benefit. For practical and ethical reasons, clearly distinguishing between research performed by public health practitioners and agencies (e.g., public health research) and public health practice is critical. This is particularly important as Bamberg [32] notes that, when the voices of caring and research are misconstrued as the voice of curing, there are real implications. Figure 1.1 designates the many relationships between public health practice and research.

## 1.6   Public Health Practice: Then, Now, and in the Future

Public health as practiced today has been shaped by many different forces. These include diseases and other health threats, history, science, social values, and the role of government [33]. Health threats have always challenged human populations; nearly all of the diseases that have wreaked havoc on society over the centuries are still with us today, including tuberculosis, cholera, malaria, yellow fever, and AIDS. Presented below are highlights of select public health practice milestones over time.

## 1.7   From Pre-history to the Hippocratic Traditions and Public Health Practice

Recent presentations of historical evidence note that from the beginnings of the civilization in the late fourth millennium BC until the Persian invasion of 525 BC, Egyptian medical practice, one of the earliest, went largely unchanged and included simple non-invasive surgery, setting of bones, dentistry, and an extensive set of pharmacopeia [34]. Others have noted that Egyptian medical thought influenced later traditions, including those of the Greeks. Relatively recent works relives the historical observations made around 440 BC. A book chapter authored by Jounna claims that the Greek historian Herodotus visited Egypt around 440 BC and wrote extensively of his observations of their medicinal practice [35]. Hippocrates (the "father of medicine") and later Galen studied at the temple of Amenhotep and acknowledged the contribution of ancient Egyptian medicine to Greek medicine, Said notes [36].

However, dominant medical literature attributes the principles of modern medicine to Greece under the influence of Hippocrates (460–375 BC). New, albeit restricted in influence, philosophies dispelling the divine nature of disease began to emerge under the Hippocrates [37]. The school of Hippocrates maintained that disease was a naturally occurring event, focused on patient treatment, emphasized prevention and lifestyle, and was guided by an ethical code [38]. The teachings of Hippocrates recognized that health and disease were affected by season and the quality of environments. It assumed that the body was made up of four fluids or humors, blood, black bile, yellow bile, and phlegm, which mirrored the four essential elements of the physical universe: fire, earth, air, and water. The body was considered healthy if all four humors were correctly balanced [37]. A Hippocratic text, On Airs, Waters, and Places, may be the first epidemiologic attempt to describe human disease and its environmental determinants [39]. The text provided a theoretical basis for the classification of disease as endemic (persistent) and epidemic (occurs occasionally affecting a number of people) [40]. The essential elements described in the text can still find meaning in the fight against public health challenges of today [41].

Post Hippocrates, Galen (c. 129–200 AD) continued promoting the Hippocratic Corpus by asserting that the causes of health and disease which produced imbalance of humors within the body could be described as "natural" (innate), "non-natural" (environmental), and "preternatural" (pathological) [40]. Galen showed through experimentation that blood was the primary humor, through which all disease could be controlled or treated [40, 42]. He proposed that adhering to protocols of diet, exercise, personal hygiene, behavior, and emotions resulted in healthy humoral balance [43]. He advocated that six determinants of health, "air and environment," "food and drink," "motion and rest," "sleep and wake," "retention and evacuation," and "passions of the mind" (emotions), should be successfully manipulated to ensure good health [40, 43]. These have endured the test of time as guidebooks of public health practice of the twentieth century feature same or similar recommendations.

Quite recently, a contribution from [44] focusing on "Medicine in Africa," in a book that examined medicine in non-western cultures, is relevant. They note that health and healing practices in sub-Saharan Africa have evolved over three millennia in constant interchange with those of other world regions. However, through the influence of Islamic medicine ("prophetic medicine"), notions of health and healing to Africa drifted significantly and were later got seriously decimated by Christian faith healing. All these perspectives coexist in the twenty-first century with African perspectives on health, sickness, and healing.

## 1.8   Public Health Practice During the Middle Ages

During the middle ages, the Church, which had authority over Europe, played a prominent role in public health administration [37]. Under the influence of Christianity, institutionalized charity expanded, providing various forms of care and shelter for the poor and sick. By the end of the sixth century, institutions (hospitals) which provided care to the sick, the leprous, and poor had become widespread. This later spread to the Islamic world too [40]. Of note, such institutionalized healthcare provisioning associated with religion is still relevant today.

Of many health challenges during this period, the waves of the Bubonic Plague stand out. Also referred to as the Black Death, the Bubonic Plague pandemic occurred in Afro-Eurasia from 1346 to 1353. It documented as the most fatal pandemic recorded in human history, causing the death of 75–200 million people in Eurasia and North Africa, peaking in Europe. It was believed to be caused by "miasma" (bad air), and hence its treatment reflected this belief. Benefiting from hindsight, the Bubonic Plague was caused by a bacterium and transmitted via the fleas of rodents. The management of the plague introduced antecedents of public health methods of disease surveillance and quarantine – victims had to report to authorities, and travelers and merchandise were isolated for 40 days or cordoned off with physical barriers when suspected of exposure to the disease [37, 45]. Disease surveillance, quarantine, and isolation remain central to the fight against modern-day public health challenges [46].

## 1.9   The Industrial Revolution and Public Health Practice

As the economies shifted toward an industrial society, people moved away from rural agricultural areas, and populations became concentrated in cities. The Industrial Revolution saw the issue of public health become a matter at the heart of government policy [47]. A rising population coupled with poor housing, poor working conditions, deficiencies in urban utilities, amenities, and neglect in public health provision led to conditions in urban areas becoming awful [45, 48]. All of such have implications of this on disease acquisition and transmission. For instance, between 1801 and 1841, the population of London doubled to nearly two million, and slums quickly grew to bear the weight of the rapid increase in people contributing to severe outbreaks of diseases such as smallpox, cholera, typhoid, and tuberculosis [49]. The cholera epidemic of 1831 and 1832 drew attention to the deplorable state of environmental sanitation in the industrial cities. New York in the 1860s was a similar story with filth and garbage accumulation at unprecedented levels linked to smallpox and cases of typhus (Committee for the Study of the Future of Public Health Services, 1988) [50].

## 1.10  Public Health Practice in the Nineteenth Century: The Emergence of Bacteriology and Contribution of Epidemiology to Public Health

According a report by the Institute of Medicine, the mid-to-late nineteenth century ushered in an era where major communicable diseases were brought under control through science applied to public health. Between 1848 and 1854, a series of outbreaks of cholera ravaged London with devastating consequences [50]. It's widely recorded that Dr. John Snow, an English epidemiologist, investigated the outbreak and was able to link the epidemic to one water source – the Broad Street Pump. When the pump handle was removed, the disease incidence drastically decreased [51]. Although the discovery of the causative agent of cholera, *Vibrio cholerae*, occurred decades later, the work of John Snow is seen as a classic example of applied epidemiology which is studied to this day [51]. Given its focus and its ultimate goal, epidemiology is instrumental to the discipline in public health. It has helped and continues to enlighten the world about the etiology of disease/ill health and their distribution in populations – brining clarity as to when it occurs, establishing more acceptable methods of measuring its risk factors and outcomes. "In its very name, epidemiology, lie the Greek words disease, people, and study (epi: upon; demos: people; logos: study), which are translated as the study of 'what falls on the population,' understood to be death, disease outbreak, possibly in endemic, epidemic, or pandemic form" [52]. Many definitional perspectives of the term exist in public health. The following is a sampling from the long list. Beaglehole defines epidemiology as "the study of the occurrence and distribution of diseases and other health related conditions in populations" [53]. Professor Last extends Professor Beaglehole's – adding to "the distribution and determinants of health-related states or events," its application to the control of health problems [54]. A leading Ghanaian epidemiologist, John Gyapong unpacked the concept to lay public, noting that, as a public health discipline, epidemiology attempts to address both individual and collective questions such as "why has this condition afflicted me (us), in this way, at this time?"

French chemist and microbiologist Louis Pasteur, and German scientist Robert Koch, led the advances into bacteriology. Pasteur demonstrated the process of microbial anaerobic fermentation, leading to the awareness of germs and establishment of the germ theory – the idea that certain microorganisms are responsible for causing many specific diseases [55]. In 1881 Pasteur established the principle of protective vaccines and thus stimulated an interest in the mechanisms of immunity [55]. Koch, in the process of discovering the causes of anthrax, cholera, and tuberculosis (1882–1883), developed four criteria designed to assess whether a microorganism causes a disease. These criteria, also known as Koch's postulates, must be fulfilled to establish a causal relationship between a parasite and a disease [56]. These criteria are largely relevant today in epidemiology.

Other notable discoveries during this period are as follows: English surgeon Joseph Lister developed concepts of antiseptic surgery, and English physician

Ronald Ross identified the mosquito as the carrier of malaria. Thus, modern public health and preventive medicine owe much to the early medical entomologists and bacteriologists. The identification of bacteria and the development of interventions such as immunization had a profound impact on public health. For the first time, it was known that diseases had single, specific causes and both the environment and people could be the agents of disease. Thus, public agencies that till then had been focusing on sanitary measures refined their activities and expanded into laboratory science and epidemiology. Public health was now inclusive of both environmental sanitation and individual health and guided by engineers, chemists, biologists, and physicians [49].

## 1.11    Public Health Practice in the Twentieth Century

At the beginning of the twentieth century, there were few effective medical treatments for disease, but improved public health standards resulted in reduced mortality and increased longevity.

The modern era of public health from the 1960s has brought a new focus on noninfectious disease epidemiology and prevention. Studies on epidemiology of risk factors of diseases and their impact on health studies have yielded important results for prevention of some chronic diseases (e.g., of the impact of diet and smoking on cardiovascular diseases). As a result, modern public health has through health promotion and advocacy played a significant role in mortality and morbidity reduction for a spectrum of diseases [51]. The twentieth century saw great achievements in global public health. In the United States, the CDC estimated that the average American gained an extra 25 years on their lifespan due to public health advancement [57]. A series of publications in 1999 reviewed ten great achievements of public health in the century, as shown in Table 1.1.

The milestones of public health in the twentieth century is not complete without the landmark report issued by the Institute of Medicine (IOM) in 1988 entitled *The Future of Public Health* [50]. This report examined the state of public health practice in the 1980s and concluded that the public health system was in a state of "disarray" and that it required a major reengineering effort. The report proposed that governmental public health be organized around three broad functions: assessment, policy development, and assurance. Basically, these translate into identifying what should be done (assessment), what will be done (policy development), and achieving those ends (assurance) [58]. Identifying what should be done comes from a comprehensive and broadly participatory assessment of needs and assets and involves both science and values. Determining what will be done recognizes that not all needs can be met and that some needs are more important than others. Achieving agreed-upon ends involves evidence-based decisions about what works and what doesn't in a particular setting and about who needs to be involved in community interventions [58]. – the authors of the second IOM Report noted [59].

**Table 1.1**  Ten great public health achievements (1900–1999)

| |
|---|
| Vaccination: the widespread use of vaccines has helped in the eradication of diseases such as smallpox and poliomyelitis in the Americas and control of others such as measles, rubella, tetanus, and diphtheria |
| Motor-vehicle safety: improvements in vehicular and road engineering, along with increased personal safety measures (e.g., increased use of safety belts and decreased drinking and driving) have contributed to large reductions in motor-vehicle-related deaths |
| Safer workplaces: since 1980, safer workplaces have resulted in a reduction of approximately 40% in the rate of fatal occupational injuries |
| Control of infectious diseases: due to improvements in environmental sanitation and water, infections such as typhoid and cholera, which had a high mortality in earlier centuries, have been significantly reduced. Antimicrobial therapy has also been a cornerstone in public health efforts to successfully control diseases like tuberculosis and sexually transmitted diseases (STDs) |
| Decline in deaths from coronary heart disease and stroke: since 1972, coronary heart disease mortality rates have decreased 51%. This can be attributed to improvements in risk factor modification, blood pressure control, and better access to treatment |
| Safer and healthier foods: programs aimed at improving nutritional content of food and decrease contamination have made food safer and healthier and significantly reduced major nutritional deficiency diseases such as rickets |
| Healthier mothers and babies: since 1900, infant mortality has decreased 90%, and maternal mortality has decreased 99% in the United States. This is due to improved nutrition and hygiene, availability of antibiotics, better access to healthcare, and technological advances in maternal and neonatal medicine |
| Family planning and contraceptive services: family planning has provided many health and socio-economic benefits for women. Examples of benefits include smaller family size and longer birth spacing; fewer infant, child, and maternal deaths; and the use of barrier contraceptives to prevent HIV and STD transmission |
| Fluoridation of drinking water: between 1945 and 1999, an estimated 144 million persons got access to fluoridized water in the United States. Fluoridation has played an important role in the downward trends of tooth decay and tooth loss |
| Recognition of tobacco use as a health hazard: public health anti-smoking campaigns have successfully reduced the prevalence of smoking among adults via behavior modification and environmental controls, averting, and millions of smoking-related deaths |

Source: Bunker et al. [57]

## 1.12   Public Health Practice in the Twenty-First Century and Beyond

Although important achievements have been made over the years – as outlined above, challenges remain. The twenty-first-century public health challenges are enormous, as there are opportunities. The challenges include an aging population, unhealthy lifestyles, the burden of increased mortality and morbidity from non-communicable diseases (NCDs), the rapid spread of infectious pathogens and the potential for global pandemics, mass migration and conflicts, mental health issues, and the health impacts of climate change and environmental pollution [60]. Undoubtedly, today's public health practice faces many challenges. There are scores of continuing health problems (such as cancer, injuries, AIDS), emerging ones (such as COVID-19, climate change, obesity), re-emerging ones (such as tuberculosis), and a slew of news issues on the public health practice agenda. While health status has never been better (as measured by life expectancy and infant mortality), the gains have not been shared equally by all segments of the population. The current increasing wealth in certain section of the population, and at the same time increasing poverty, smacks of humanity's failure and thus a  public health failure. These unacceptable realities challenge public health practitioners' core values of realizing public health's dream of social justice and creating a health system organized around health. To meet the challenges, public health practice will have to relearn the lessons of its past and move to expand its circle to include new sectors of society at every level of government – namely, more community partners and stakeholders and a more involved citizenry.

There are opportunities – technology and people. Some have argued that the future of public health practice lies in these technologies, in precision public health, but also social public health. Precision public health can be simply defined as "providing the right intervention to the right population at the right time" [61]. More accurate methods to study the interactions between biological and genetic factors with personal, environmental, and social determinants of health could allow better assessment of population health and development of policies and targeted programs for preventing disease [61, 62]. Current and future opportunities for advancing precision public health should include priority actions such as improving data integration, transdisciplinary partnerships, enhancing public health surveillance and tracking, focusing on "precision prevention" and early detection, and incorporating initiatives that address health equity [61, 63, 64].

However, given the multi-scaled challenges of public health, public health practice of today and in the future must recognize the critical relevance of social public health. Globally, social determinants of health – the link between people's health and the social conditions in which they live and work – have been highlighted as integral to reduce health inequities and improve health outcomes. The WHO in March 2005 launched the Commission on Social Determinants of Health (CSDH), to assist countries to centralize health equity in all policies and promote evidence-based practices that address these social determinants of health [65]. Current public health approaches are emphasizing the need to shift health away from being disease-focused to health events or people-focused. Focusing on these social determinants is integral for governments to meet their development goals, reduce health inequalities, promote population health, and create and sustain economically viable societies [65]. Nearly a decade later, [66] highlights some of the public health consequences of the chasm between the biomedical and social sciences that is an artifact of our system of professional education. It underscores the need to bridge the divide in order to improve the delivery of public health services. A renewed public health must address social, cultural, and economic differentials that deny the public the enjoyment of their basic rights. It must also promote justice (politically, economically, socially, and culturally). It must address what West and Marteau referred to us "commercial determinants of health" (factors that influence health which stem from the profit motive) and what Gostin et al. termed "legal determinants of health" [67, 68]. They articulate the crucial role of law in achieving global public health through legal instruments, legal capacities, and institutional reforms, as well as a firm commitment to the rule of law.

For all of these to be realized, the ultimate beneficiaries – the publics of public health – must be in a position to contribute meaningfully and sufficiently. Even with precision public health, the practice of public health in the twenty-first century and in the future will not be effective without true engagements with the publics of public health. Tools such as advocacy, community engagement and empowerment, and scholar activism and processes such as community mobilization, sensitization, and countering political controversies, misinformation, disinformation, and conspiracy theories remain relevant, particularly in social public health.

**The Book**

Responding to public health challenges at the global and local levels can give rise to an array of tensions. To assure sustainable public health, these tensions need to be meaningfully balanced. This book enunciates the many dimensions of national-level responses to AIDS. Calling out glaring neglects, the book makes a bold recommendation for the destabilization of the naturalness with which national AIDS responses ignore the socio-political and medico-ethical dimensions of AIDS. The case made is grounded in the philosophy of social public health. Packed with relevant conceptual, philosophical, and methodological perspectives, the book makes a compelling read for a broad spectrum of people: public policy, bioethics, and social sciences, professionals/scholars, and students of those fields. Also, public health economists, lay politicians, and civil society organizations advocating for health equity will find the book useful. The book is timely. It is written at a time when public health actors are repositioning themselves to be competent users of not only pharmaceutic vaccines but also social vaccines.

Each of the seven chapters that follow this introductory chapter is summarized below.

*Chapter 2* presents the public health approaches to HIV and AIDS. Beginning from the early days of AIDS, the chapter discusses the conceptualization of HIV (including AIDS) as a public health emergency of international concern. The chapter describes the global response to HIV – examining the application of cardinal public health principles to curbing AIDS in different contexts and the achievements of traditional public health practice measures (including surveillance, testing, the counting and reporting AIDS cases, and deaths) as well as relatively recent innovations (including combination prevention measures, treatment as prevention). Also discussed are the prospects and challenges of efforts aimed at eliminating HIV. The chapter argues that public health response to HIV will not chalk durable success without addressing old challenges such as AIDS denialism, misinformation, and conspiracy theories but also new and disinformation and AIDS infodemia.

*Chapter 3* identifies and discusses HIV/AIDS countermeasures. Such measures include traditional HIV prevention efforts of abstinence, fidelity, use of condoms, AIDS prevention measures such as treatment with antiretroviral medications (ARVs), nutrition interventions, as well as social care and psychosocial support. Donning a social public health lens, the chapter debates the relative importance of these interventions – emphasizing not just whether the interventions work but for whom and under what circumstances. Through such analysis, the chapter responds to the questions of "which interventions count? Which do not? And why not?" The chapter concludes with a recommendation to ensure meaningful integration of all relevant interventions into what is currently predominantly a medical response.

*Chapter 4* examines medical but also cultural constructions of access and the evolving discourses on access to life-saving AIDS medications. It traces the discourses from the era of frank absence to AIDS medications to rationing of same and to the current era of "test and treat." Drawing on extant texts on access in general and access to AIDS medications in particular, the chapter identifies gaps in the current notion of access. The chapter argues that the current global aspirational goal of "treat all"/"test and treat" requires a nuanced understanding of the multiple notions of access and their variegated political economies.

*Chapter 5* provides an analysis of how enactment and enforcement of rights-limiting policies, regulations, or legislations not only limit rights but also amplify risks and vulnerabilities to HIV in key and general populations. Drawing on prevailing rights discourses and pedagogy, the chapter offers two approaches to responding to the syndemic of HIV and rights violations. The proposed approaches are grounded in abolitionist and instrumentalist doctrines.

*Chapter 6* discusses data from an exercise that examined how responsive Ghana's National AIDS policy documents/guidelines are to social, cultural, political, and ethical contexts. The chapter highlights key measures to developing and implementing national AIDS response policies that do not lose sight of how policy insensitivities but also how social forces and other structural barriers affect realization of health. Although focused on Ghana's AIDS response guidelines, the analysis presented in the chapter enables identification of gaps in similar national public health policies.

*Chapter 7* – the final chapter of the book – illustrates efforts by a multidisciplinary team of researchers and practitioners (public health professionals, clinicians, social workers) to engage relevant actors to adopt and integrate social public health approaches into Ghana's national response to HIV/AIDS. The chapter shares the implementation approaches and lessons from the Consortium. The initiative calls attention to the need to demystify public health practice and to destabilize age-old public health orthodoxies (where privileged "certificated" few, usually with biomedical background, are mandated to assure public health). Lessons from the initiative show that multiple actors (both expert and lay) are required to execute specific tasks and play unique roles.

# References

1. Laar A, Ganle J, Owusu A, Tenkorang E, Tuakli-Wosornu YA, Soyiri I, Okyerefo M, Senah K. Representing health: an afrocentric Perspective from Ghana. In: Makanga PT, editor. Practicing health geography: the African context. Cham: Springer; 2021. p. 93–104.
2. Sigerist HE. A history of medicine (Early Greek, Hindu and Persian medicine), vol. II. New York: Oxford University Press; 1961.
3. Tountas Y. The historical origins of the basic concepts of health promotion and education: the role of ancient Greek philosophy and medicine. Health Promot Int. 2009;24(2):185–92.
4. Ergil KV, Ergfl M, Furst P, Gordon N, Janzen J, Sobo E, Sparrowe L. Ancient healing: unlocking the mysteries of health and healing through the ages. Lincolnwood Publications. ISBN-10: 785324313; 1997. p. 68–95.
5. Bloom BL. The "medical model," miasma theory, and community mental health. Community Ment Health J. 1965;1(4):333–8.
6. Sterner CS. A brief history of miasmic theory. Bull Hist Med. 1948;22:747.
7. Brack A. The molecular origins of life: assembling pieces of the puzzle. Cambridge: Cambridge University Press; 1998.
8. Tyndall J. Fragments of science (Vol. 2). New York: P. F. Collier. Chapters IV, XII (1876), XIII (1878). Retrieved from https://archive.org/details/fragmenoscien02tyndrich. 1905.
9. Karamanou M, Panayiotakopoulos G, Tsoucalas G, Kousoulis AA, Androutsos G. From miasmas to germs: a historical approach to theories of infectious disease transmission. Infez Med. 2012;20(1):58–62.
10. WHO. Constitution of the World Health Organization. Basic documents. Geneva. 1948.
11. Boddington P, Räisänen U. Theoretical and practical issues in the definition of health: insights from aboriginal Australia. J Med Philos. 2009;2009:49–67.
12. King M, Smith A, Gracey M. Indigenous health part 2: the underlying causes of the health gap. Lancet. 2009;374(9683):76–85.
13. Thiessen K, Haworth-Brockman M, Stout R, Moffitt P, Gelowitz J, Schneider J, Demczuk L. Indigenous perspectives on wellness and health in Canada: study protocol for a scoping review. Syst Rev. 2020;9(1):1–6.
14. Bacchetta L, Visioli F, Cappelli G, Caruso E, Martin G, Nemeth E, Bacchetta G, Bedini G, Wezel A, van Asseldonk T. A manifesto for the valorization of wild edible plants. J Ethnopharmacol. 2016;191:180–7.
15. Asare M, Danquah SA. The African belief system and the patient's choice of treatment from existing health models-the case of Ghana. Acta Psychopathol. 2017;3(4):49.
16. Gessert C, Waring S, Bailey-Davis L, Conway P, Roberts M, VanWormer J. Rural definition of health: a systematic literature review. BMC Public Health. 2015;15(1):1–14.
17. Omonzejele PF. African concepts of health, disease, and treatment: an ethical inquiry. Explore (NY). 2008;4(2):120–6.
18. Oti-Boadi M. Exploring the lived experiences of mothers of children with intellectual disability in Ghana. SAGE Open. 2017;7(4):2158244017745578.
19. Harrell JA, Baker EL. The essential services of public health. Leadership Pub Health. 1994;3(3):27–31.
20. Dowdle WR, Hopkins DR. The eradication of infectious diseases: report of the Dahlem workshop on the eradication of infections diseases. Chichester: Wiley; 1998. p. 218.
21. CDC P. Recommendations of the international task force for disease eradication. Morb Mortal Wkly Rep. 1993;42:1–38.
22. Thacker SB, Berkelman RL. Public health surveillance in the United States. Epidemiol Rev. 1988;10(1):164–90.
23. Declich S, Carter AO. Public health surveillance: historical origins, methods and evaluation. Bull World Health Organ. 1994;72(2):285.
24. Galva JE, Atchison C, Levey S. Public health strategy and the police powers of the state. Public Health Rep. 2005;120(1 suppl):20–7.

25. Pennsylvania General Assembly, Local Government Commission. What is the "police power"? Pennsylvania Legislator's Municipal Deskbook. http://www.lgc.state.pa.us/deskbook03/Issues17.pdf. 2003.
26. Gostin LO, Wiley LF. Governmental public health powers during the COVID-19 pandemic: stay-at-home orders, business closures, and travel restrictions. JAMA. 2020;323(21):2137–8.
27. Otto JL, Holodniy M, DeFraites RF. Public health practice is not research. Am J Public Health. 2014;104(4):596–602.
28. Getting VA, Ryder CF. The theory and practice of public health. N Engl J Med. 1953;249(9):354–61.
29. Levine R. Boundaries between research involving human subjects and accepted and routine professional practices. In: Bogomolny RL, editor. HumaN n er nentatio. Dallas: Southern Methodist UniversityPress; 1976. p. 3–10.
30. Appelbaum PS, Roth LH, Lidz C. The therapeutic misconception: informed consent in psychiatric research. Int J Law Psychiatry. 1982;5(3–4):319–29.
31. Pentz RD, White M, Harvey RD, Farmer ZL, Liu Y, Lewis C, Dashevskaya O, Owonikoko T, Khuri FR. Therapeutic misconception, misestimation, and optimism in participants enrolled in phase 1 trials. Cancer. 2012;118(18):4571–8.
32. Bamberg M, Budwig N. Therapeutic misconceptions: when the voices of caring and research are misconstrued as the voice of curing. Ethics Behav. 1992;2(3):165–84.
33. Encyclopedia of Public Health. Retrieved October 25, 2021 from Encyclopedia.com. https://www.encyclopedia.com/education/encyclopedias-almanacs-transcripts-and-maps/practice-public-health
34. Bryan CP, Smith GE. Ancient Egyptian medicine: the papyrus ebers. Chicago: Ares Publishers; 1930.
35. Jouanna J, Allies N. Egyptian medicine and Greek medicine. In: Greek medicine from Hippocrates to Galen. Brill; 2012. p. 1–20.
36. Said GZ. Orthopaedics in the dawn of civilisation, practices in ancient Egypt. Int Orthop. 2014;38(4):905–9.
37. Leiyu Shi. Novick & Morrow's Public Health Administration: principles for population-based management. Jones & Bartlett Learning. https://books.google.com.gh/books?id=-IiOAwAAQBAJ&pg=PA11&dq=chapter+2+Historical+Developments+in+Public+Health+and+the+21st+Century&hl=en&sa=X&ved=2ahUKEwiU3fuw_IfxAhUZ7eAKHcfgDYoQ6wEwBnoECAMQAQ#v=onepage&q=chapter%202&f=false. 2013.
38. Dubovsky H. The Jewish contribution to medicine Part I. Biblical and Talmudic times to the end of the 18th century. S Afr Med J. 1989;76(1):26–8.
39. Rhodes P. Public health | definition, history, & facts | Britannica. Britannica. https://www.britannica.com/topic/public-health. 2005.
40. Porter D. Health, civilization and the state: a history of public health from ancient to modern times. London: Routledge; 2005.
41. Harmer A, Eder B, Gepp S, Leetz A, van de Pas R. WHO should declare climate change a public health emergency. BMJ. 2020;368:m797.
42. Hajar R. The air of history: early medicine to Galen (part I). Heart Views. 2012;13(3):120.
43. Berryman JW. Motion and rest: Galen on exercise and health. Lancet. 2012;380(9838):210–1.
44. Janzen JM, Green EC. Medicine in Africa. In: Selin H, editor. Encyclopaedia of the history of science, technology, and medicine in non-western cultures. Dordrecht: Springer; 2008. p. 1493–508.
45. Boston University School of Public Health. A brief history of public health. BU Office of Teaching & Digital Learning, 2015. https://sphweb.bumc.bu.edu/otlt/mph-modules/ph/publichealthhistory/publichealthhistory_print.html. 2015.
46. WHO. Public health surveillance for COVID-19. Beyond Anthrax, 2019(August), 253–278. WHO/2019-nCoV/SurveillanceGuidance/2020.7; 2020.
47. Public health in the industrail age. Sociol Rev 1919; a11(1):49–61.

48. Bynum WF, Porter R. Living and dying in London: introduction. Med Hist Suppl. 1991;1991(11):vii–xviii.
49. Rhodes P. Public health: national developments in the 18th and 19th centuries. In: Encyclopedia Britannica. https://www.britannica.com/topic/public-health/National-developments-in-the-18th-and-19th-centuries#ref412440. 2015.
50. Health IoMUCftSotFoP. The future of public health. Washington: National Academies Press (US); 1988. 3, A history of the public health system. Available from: https://www.ncbi.nlm.nih.gov/books/NBK218224/. 1988.
51. Tulchinsky TH, Varavikova EA. A history of public health. New Pub Health. 2014:1–42.
52. Azevedo MJ. Public health in Africa: THEOreTICAL framework. In: Historical perspectives on the state of health and health systems in Africa, vol. I. Cham: Springer; 2017. p. 1–77.
53. Beaglehole R, Bonita R, Kjellström T. Basic epidemiology. Geneva: World Health Organization; 1993.
54. Last JM. International Epidemiological Association. A dictionary of epidemiology. New York: Oxford University Press; 2001.
55. Silver GA. A history of public health. Am J Pub Health Nations Health. 1958;48(7):944–5.
56. Segre JA. What does it take to satisfy koch's postulates two centuries later? Microbial genomics and propionibacteria acnes. J Investig Dermatol. 2013;133(9):2141–2.
57. Bunker JP, Frazier HS, Mosteller F. Improving health: measuring effects of medical care. Milbank Q. 1994;72(2):225–58.
58. Practice of Public Health. Encyclopedia of public health. Retrieved April 25, 2022 from Encyclopedia.com: https://www.encyclopedia.com/education/encyclopedias-almanacs-transcripts-and-maps/practice-public-health
59. Institute of Medicine Committee on Using Performance Monitoring to Improve Community Health. Improving health in the community: a role for performance monitoring. Washington, DC: National Academy Press; 1997.
60. World Health Organisation. Facing the future: opportunities and challenges for 21st-century public health in implementing the Sustainable Development Goals and the Health 2020 policy framework. June 2018, 1–19. http://www.euro.who.int/__data/assets/pdf_file/0003/374052/180278-public-health-future-eng.pdf?ua=1. 2018.
61. Khoury MJ, Iademarco MF, Riley WT. Precision public health for the era of precision medicine. Am J Prev Med. 2016;50(3):398.
62. Velmovitsky PE, Bevilacqua T, Alencar P, Cowan D, Morita PP. Convergence of precision medicine and public health into precision public health: toward a big data perspective. Front Public Health. 2021;9(305)
63. Olstad DL, McIntyre L. Reconceptualising precision public health. BMJ Open. 2019;9(9):e030279.
64. Roberts MC, Fohner AE, Landry L, Olstad DL, Smit AK, Turbitt E, Allen CG. Advancing precision public health using human genomics: examples from the field and future research opportunities. Genome Med. 2021;13(1):97.
65. World Health Organization. Commission on social determinants of health. 2006.
66. Giles-Vernick T, Webb JL Jr. Global health in Africa: historical perspectives on disease control. Athens: Ohio University Press; 2013.
67. Gostin LO, Monahan JT, Kaldor J, DeBartolo M, Friedman EA, Gottschalk K, Kim SC, Alwan A, Binagwaho A, Burci GL. The legal determinants of health: harnessing the power of law for global health and sustainable development. Lancet. 2019;393(10183):1857–910.
68. West R, Marteau T. Commentary on Casswell (2013): the commercial determinants of health. Addiction. 2013;108(4):686–7.

# Chapter 2
# Public Health Approaches to HIV and AIDS

## 2.1 Introduction

In 1981, I was too young to have heard of, let alone read about acquired immunodeficiency syndrome (AIDS). There was no such lexicon as human immunodeficiency virus (HIV) in medical or public health dictionaries then. Indeed, most adults, irrespective of the region of the world that they were, had never heard about AIDS. As Dr. Everett Koop *of Blessed Memory* put it, "…the handful of scientists (in the US and Europe) who knew about the condition didn't even know what to call it" [1]. As far are the dominant "formal" public health literature on the subject is concerned, it all started at about June 1981. The Centers for Disease Control and Prevention (CDC) of the United States published its first report of what was to become the AIDS epidemic. It concerned five "previously healthy" gay men who were admitted to Los Angeles hospitals with a very rare form of pneumonia. By the time the report had been published, two of the men had died. The other three died shortly thereafter – Koop [1] narrates. A couple of weeks later, the US public health service published a report that about two dozens of young homosexual men had been recently diagnosed as having Kaposi's sarcoma (a cancerous condition rarely found among young men). This nameless novel condition was given a somewhat awkward "name" – the "acquired immune deficiency syndrome" – when it was recognized that all who had these conditions were immune suppressed. For a short time, some people called it gay-related immune deficiency (GRID). Later when cases were discovered among non-gay persons, the name reverted to AIDS [1]. The early years of the AIDS epidemic were filled with uncertainty, fear, and confusion. Reports of other similar cases in other parts of the world brought more attention to the scientific community. During those early days of AIDS, scientists did not only struggle to identify what caused the illness, what to call it, and how it was transmitted but also how to "deal" with those who had the disease, those who were exposed to the disease, and those who were perceived to be the reservoirs or vectors of the disease.

And so, ethicists and human rights advocates were made busy by AIDS as were epidemiologists and infectious disease experts. As subject experts struggled with the epidemic of AIDS, the epidemic of stigma associated with the condition spread like wildfire during the *Harmattan* season. And so social scientists got busy too. At a point, even economists got busy – when it finally dawned on the world that AIDS was not just another infectious disease but a broader developmental challenge. The concept of historical presentism permits me to write now (in 2021) that the two reasons why it took a while for public health authorities to get a handle on AIDS were, first, the relatively few trained clinicians and researchers familiar with the novel disease and, second, the fact that the first patients with those conditions were homosexual men, most of whom patronized physicians and clinics that were more understanding of the so-called gay lifestyle. As Koop aptly describes it, in making a reasonable choice, these men effectively placed themselves outside mainstream public health response and, therefore, were more difficult to know, to reach, and to help [1]. This also stymied the global public health response in other ways. For instance, the world's first public health priority – stopping further transmission of the AIDS virus – became mired in the homosexual politics, and it would seem to me this has endured. Over 40 years following the emergence of AIDS, the gay label has and continues to contribute to the apathetic response from political leaders and the community at large. Although AIDS literacy has markedly improved, some still see it as God's retribution to those who practiced the gay lifestyle and drug users. It is instructive to note that the global public health response lost a great deal of precious time because of this and therefore lives.

Unknown to the rest of the world, doctors in some African countries had seen a rise in opportunistic infections and wasting a decade earlier [2]. A year later, French and American scientists identified the causative organism, which also went through a series of nomenclature until they finally settled for what we know as human immunodeficiency virus (HIV). Notwithstanding the discovery of the causative agent of AIDS, and appreciation of its modes of transmission, acquiring HIV in the decades that followed was synonymous to a death sentence. Not only was there no known treatment for the virus, the stigma associated with HIV diagnosis was itself lethal. And so those early days of AIDS, and to some extent, till now would be filled with mystery, suspicion, stigma, discrimination, and fear of the unknown. Before examining the global response to AIDS, I summarize here some cardinal milestones in the global response to HIV.

From those small beginnings in the 1980s, what started as an outbreak metamorphosed into an epidemic mushroomed into a Public Health Emergency of International Concern (PHEIC) and then into a full-fledged pandemic and is now endemic in several countries. Readers may find expatiation on these levels of disease concepts relevant.

The CDC [3] describes the amount of a particular disease (or a health event) that is usually present in a community as the baseline or endemic level of the disease. This level is not necessarily the desired level, which may in fact be zero, but rather is the observed level. In the absence of intervention and assuming that the level is not high enough to deplete the pool of susceptible persons, the disease may continue to occur at this level indefinitely. While some diseases are so rare in a given population that a single case warrants an epidemiologic investigation (e.g., rabies, plague, polio), other diseases occur more commonly so that only deviations from the norm warrant investigation. Occasionally, the amount of disease in a community rises above the expected level, and such levels are described as an outbreak. An epidemic, on the other hand, is defined by the WHO as "the occurrence in a community or region of cases of an illness, specific health-related behavior, or other health-related events clearly in excess of normal expectancy." As you would have noticed, an outbreak carries the same definition of epidemic but is often used for a more limited geographic area. The WHO defines PHEIC as an extraordinary event which is determined to constitute a public health risk to other states through the international spread of disease and to potentially require a coordinated international response [4]. This definition designates a public health crisis of potentially global reach and implies a situation that is "serious, sudden, unusual, or unexpected," which may necessitate immediate international action. States have a legal duty to respond promptly to a PHEIC. Pandemic, the most serious classification of the disease level, refers to an epidemic that has spread over several countries or continents, usually affecting a large number of people, thus an epidemic occurring globally. Politically, it is only the WHO who is mandated to declare a disease or a public health challenge as a PHEIC or a pandemic.

A declaration of a pandemic obviously has public health response implications but also political implications. Throughout history, the word pandemic has been used to trigger collective global action against a large-scale epidemic. And so, HIV was declared one. Thus, reigning for 40 years, the HIV pandemic is arguably the longest raging pandemic in recent human history and the fifth deadliest from ancient Rome to modern era [5]. During the period, a lot has been learned about the pandemic. As Everett Koop put it, "we have come from not knowing what AIDS was, not knowing the causative agent of the disease. We identified the virus, named it and renamed it. We identified antibodies to the AIDS virus and developed a screening test on the basis of the detection of these antibodies. We learned how to kill the virus in blood products –making blood transfusion safer. We have even sequenced the genome of the virus." Those who have lived through the very troubling days of the HIV pandemic may be content that it is now a chronic illness with multiple effective countermeasures (including medications to treat it).

We understood the epidemiology among (various segments of the population – men, women, children, sex workers, men who have sex with men (MSM), etc.). Nevertheless, myths, conspiracy theories, and outright denialism remain and are a barrier to accessing care. The global AIDS response must meaningfully and sufficiency address these for a sustainable success. Following, I describe the global responses to HIV and the various public health approaches used.

## 2.2   The Global Public Health Response to the HIV Pandemic

At all times challenges associated with public health responses to any health challenge abound. During a pandemic, these challenges are amplified. When a pandemic is declared, international and national countermeasures, which include action to "contain, delay, mitigate" (as described in Chap. 1), usually have both positive and negative externalities.

Each of these phases of a pandemic presents unique logistical and moral conundrums to health systems and professionals. Logistically, pandemics tend to be a serious threat to the stability of health systems, imposing extraordinarily challenging and sustained demands on them, which can exceed the service capacity regarding all their available supplies and technologies or human resources. Morally, pandemics pose the enormous challenge of technical and logistical coordination but also balancing individual rights with collective rights. Navigating these require international and national guidance. That is why, the international efforts to combat HIV, which began in the first decade of the epidemic, saw the creation of the WHO's Global Programme on AIDS in 1987. The Joint United Nations Programme on HIV and AIDS (UNAIDS) was formed in 1996 to serve as the UN system's coordinating body and to help galvanize worldwide attention to AIDS.

As outlined in Table 2.1, the rapid spread of the disease and its deadly consequences all over the globe led the WHO to classify AIDS as an epidemic in 1983. By this time, cases had been reported in all continents of the earth. The first AIDS conference was convened in 1985, in Atlanta, Georgia. At that time, HIV tests had been made available and licensed for screening of blood supplies. The US Food and Drug Administration (FDA) approved the first drug for treating AIDS, azidothymidine (AZT), for use, and the Global Programme on AIDS was established by the WHO in 1987. In the early 1990s, more than 2.5 million infections of HIV/AIDS had been reported globally, and the incidence of new infections was estimated to be about 3 million in 1995. AIDS was then the leading cause of mortality in the United States among people 25 to 44 years of age [6]. A global response was indeed required to contain the epidemic. However, stakeholders who mounted the response had to also combat the stigmatization, discrimination, and denialism, stemming from the perceptions and conceptualizations of the epidemic in its infancy. In 1996, a triple-combination therapy was introduced. It proved to be very effective and started to give hope to those infected. In addition, public policy also went against the tide of social norms by educating the public about safe sex practices including abstinence, monogamous sexual relations, and condom use, leading to a surge in the sales of condoms in wealthy countries. From that time, developed countries like the United States started to see a decline in AIDS-related deaths as well as new infections for the first time. For developing countries (especially in sub-Saharan Africa who bore the brunt of the epidemic), affordable treatment and prevention interventions were yet to reach them.

The early 2000s heralded enhanced efforts by the global community to fight AIDS. A number of multilateral as well as bilateral initiatives were birthed. For

**Table 2.1**  Selected development during the first 40 years of AIDS (1981–2021)

| Year | Selected developments |
|------|----------------------|
| 1981 | CDC publishes first report of what was destined to be the AIDS epidemic (and later pandemic) first two cases of pneumonia – pneumocystis carinii pneumonia (PCP) |
| 1982 | AIDS is reported among hemophiliacs and Haitians in the United States<br>GRID is renamed AIDS<br>AIDS is linked to 5Hs: Haitians, homosexuals, heroin addicts, hookers, and hemophiliacs<br>AIDS is reported in several European countries<br>CDC's first AIDS case definition "a disease, at least moderately predictive of a defect in cell-mediated immunity, occurring in a person with no known cause for diminished resistance to that disease." Such diseases including Kaposis Sarcoma (KS), PCP, and serious opportunistic infections (fever, weight loss, persistent generalized lymphadenopathy, tuberculosis, oral candidiasis, herpes zoster) are birthed |
| 1983/84 | The causative agent of AIDS-HIV is identified by French and American Scientists, first called "lymphadenopathy-associated virus" (LAV), AID-associated retrovirus (ARV), human T-lymphotropic virus III (HTLV-III), and finally renamed human immunodeficiency virus (HIV)<br>In the same year, Western scientists become aware that AIDS is widespread in parts of Africa |
| 1985 | CDC's case definition revised to reflect AIDS that is caused by a newly identified virus<br>ELISA is licensed for clinical use<br>The First International AIDS Conference, Atlanta, Georgia, USA<br>An HIV test is licensed for screening blood supplies<br>AIDS is reported in China and has therefore been seen in all regions of the world |
| 1986 | The first AIDS case is identified in Ghana |
| 1987 | AZT is the first drug approved for treating AIDS<br>Ban on travel and immigration to the United States for HIV-positive people<br>ACT UP (AIDS Coalition to Unleash Power) holds its first demonstration on Wall Street to protest against high profit margins enjoyed by pharmaceutical companies |
| 1988 | Dr. Everett Koop as US Surgeon General plays a cardinal role in the first national AIDS campaign in the USA. Health ministers of the world meet and established December 1 as World AIDS Day |
| 1989 | Princess Diana opened Landmark AIDS Centre in the United Kingdom and gave someone diagnosed HIV positive 5 years earlier. This was the first attempt to de-stigmatize the condition by a high-profile celebrity |
| 1990 | In June, the 6th International AIDS Conference in San Francisco protested against the USA's immigration policy which stopped people with HIV from entering the country. NGOs boycotted the conference<br>In October, the FDA approved the use of zidovudine (AZT) to treat children with AIDS<br>By the end of 1990, over 307,000 AIDS cases had been officially reported with the actual number estimated to be closer to a million. Between 8 and 10 million people were thought to be living with HIV worldwide |
| 1991 | ddI – didanosine/2′,3′-dideoxyinosine approved (only two drugs, 10 years into the epidemic)<br>8–10 million people were estimated to have infected with HIV worldwide |

(continued)

**Table 2.1** (continued)

| Year | Selected developments |
|------|----------------------|
| 1992 | The 1992 International AIDS Conference scheduled to be held in Boston, USA, was moved to Amsterdam due to US immigration rules on people living with HIV<br>In May, the FDA licensed a 10-min testing kit which could be used by healthcare professionals to detect HIV-1 |
| 1993 | NIH implements new guidelines requiring that women and persons of color be included in clinical trials |
| 1994 | CDC announces that AIDS is the leading cause of death among 25–44 year olds in the United States |
| 1995 | Saquinavir, the first protease inhibitor, is approved for use (the pool of AIDS drugs were AZT, ddI, ddC, d4T, 3TC, and saquinavir) |
| 1996 | The viral load test is approved<br>Triple-combination therapy is introduced as AIDS experts advocate for hit hard, hit early<br>Highly active antiretroviral therapy (HAART), formerly known as triple-combination therapy, becomes the standard of care for AIDS |
| 1997 | The number of Americans newly diagnosed with AIDS drops for the first time since the epidemic began |
| 1998 | CDC announces that the number of American AIDS deaths dropped 47% in the previous year, largely due to the uptake of AIDS medications<br>However, side effects of HAART adherence found to be challenging to patients taking these therapies |
| 1999 | In 1999, the WHO announced that AIDS was the fourth biggest cause of death worldwide and number one killer in Africa. An estimated 33 million people were living with HIV, and 14 million people had died from AIDS since the start of the epidemic |
| 2000 | President Thabo Mbeki of South Africa voices support for AIDS dissidents<br>Nonoxynol-9, the first HIV microbicide is shown to increase the risk of HIV transmission |
| 2001 | In 2001, a United Nations General Assembly Special Session on HIV/AIDS (UNGASS) was convened, and the Global Fund was created a year after |
| 2002 | Side effects and drug resistance call "hit hard, hit early" emphasis in therapy into question<br>The Global Fund is established to boost the response to AIDS, TB, and malaria<br>Botswana begins Africa's first national AIDS treatment program |
| 2003 | AIDS drugs become more affordable for developing countries<br>The "3 by 5" campaign is launched to widen access to AIDS treatment |
| 2004 | America launches a major initiative called President's Emergency Plan for AIDS Relief (PEPFAR) to combat AIDS worldwide<br>After much hesitancy, South Africa begins to provide free antiretroviral treatment |
| 2005 | Scientists report that HIV is not a supervirus after all, as improved HIV care saved at least 2 million years of life between 1989 and 2003 |
| 2006 | The first ever one-pill fixed-dose combination for HIV therapy is approved<br>Male circumcision is shown to reduce HIV infection among heterosexual men<br>Less than 30–28% of people in developing countries who need treatment for HIV are receiving it |

(continued)

**Table 2.1** (continued)

| Year | Selected developments |
|------|----------------------|
| 2007 | About 33 million people are estimated to be living with HIV, according to revised estimates<br>A major HIV vaccine trial is halted after preliminary results show no benefit |
| 2008 | A "controversial" Swiss study claims people adhering to ARVs have a "negligibly small" risk of transmitting HIV through unprotected sex |
| 2009 | President Obama announces the lifting of the travel ban that prevents HIV-positive people from entering the United States<br>4 million people in developing and transitional countries are receiving treatment for HIV; 9.5 million are still in immediate need of treatment |
| 2010 | Concerns over issues of cardiovascular disease, bone health, liver health, and inflammatory issues drive HIV care as chronic illness<br>HIV-related travel ban is lifted in South Korea, China, and Namibia<br>The CAPRISA 004 microbicide trial is hailed a success after results show the gel reduced the risk of HIV infection by 40%. Results from a pre-exposure trial (iPrEx trial) show a reduction in HIV acquisition among men who have sex with men taking pre-exposure prophylaxis (PrEP) |
| 2011 | Results from the HPTN 052 trial show that early initiation of antiretroviral treatment reduces the risk of HIV transmission by 96% among discordant couples<br>The Global Fund announces the replacement of Round 11 with a Transitional Funding Mechanism (TFM), due to a lack of funds |
| 2012 | In 2012, the International AIDS Conference (AIDS 2012) is hosted in the United States – Washington DC – after several years, after the first Conference in 1985 |
| 2013 | Researchers describe the first "functional HIV cure" in an infant. The child was born to an HIV-infected mother and received combination antiretroviral treatment beginning 30 hours after birth. Ten months after discontinuation of treatment, the child underwent repeated standard blood tests, none of which detected HIV presence in the blood |
| 2014 | UNAIDS "Fast-Track" called for the dramatic scaling up of HIV prevention and treatment program<br>UNAIDS launched the 90-90-90 targets which aim for 90% of people living with HIV to be diagnosed, 90% of those diagnosed to be accessing antiretroviral treatment, and 90% of those accessing treatment to achieve viral suppression by 2020 |
| 2015 | WHO launched new treatment guidelines recommending that all people living with HIV receive ART regardless of CD4 count soon after diagnosis |
| 2016 | A US doctor performs the first HIV-to-HIV liver transplants. Effectiveness of new anti-HIV medication to protect women and infants demonstrated |
| 2017 | The slogan "Undetectable=Untransmutable" is launched and becomes the first defining message of the HIV response in many countries but failed to have the same impact in low-resource settings where ART monitoring is difficult |
| 2018 | There is no cure for HIV – but scientists may be getting closer<br>New research shows that an experimental HIV-1 vaccine regimen is well-tolerated and generated comparable and robust immune responses against HIV in healthy adults and rhesus monkeys. Moreover, the vaccine candidate is protected against infection with an HIV-like virus in monkeys |
| 2019 | HIV/AIDS deaths fall by one third since 2010, but experts say more could be done |

(continued)

**Table 2.1**  (continued)

| Year | Selected developments |
|------|------------------------|
| 2020 | State of 90-90-90 WHO target by 2020 Source: https://www.theglobalfund.org/en/results/ |
| 2021 | People living with HIV more likely to get sick with and die from COVID-19. New research shows that individuals living with human immunodeficiency virus (HIV) and acquired immune deficiency syndrome (AIDS) – an estimated 38 million worldwide, according to the World Health Organization – have an increased risk of SARS-CoV-2 infection and fatal outcomes from COVID-19 The "Political Declaration on HIV and AIDS: Ending Inequalities and Getting on Track to End AIDS by 2030" (document A/75/L.95), passed and adopted by the World Leaders in General Assembly https://www.un.org/press/en/2021/ga12333.doc.htm |

Source: Author's construction base on cited evidence

instance, the United States established the President's Emergency Plan for AIDS Relief (PEPFAR). These initiatives were aimed at providing the needed assistance to developing countries to curb the epidemic. Of note, only 1% of the estimated 4.1 million infected persons had received ART in sub-Saharan Africa after funds that were initially provided for that purpose were mismanaged. In 2001, a United Nations General Assembly Special Session on HIV/AIDS (UNGASS) was convened, and the Global Fund to fight AIDS, tuberculosis, and malaria was created in 2002. Recognizing insufficiency of the resource need to respond effectively, the WHO in 2003 declared the failure to provide treatment to 6 million infected people living in developing countries as a public health emergency. The WHO then announced plans to provide 3 million infected persons in developing countries with life-saving highly active antiretroviral therapy (HAART) by 2005 – the so-called 3 × 5 initiative. Negotiations for implementation of large-scale treatment programs began, and some 35 countries were prioritized for WHO support in scaling up ART [7]. For highlight of important milestones spanning 1981 to 2021, see Table 2.1.

Fast forward to 2021, the global HIV response according to the WHO [8] includes the recent endorsement at the Sixty-Ninth World Health Assembly the "Global health sector strategy on HIV for 2016–2021." The strategy includes five strategic directions that guide priority actions by countries and by the WHO over 6 years. The strategic directions are:

- Information for focused action (know your epidemic and response)
- Interventions for impact (covering the range of services needed)
- Delivering for equity (covering the populations in need of services)
- Financing for sustainability (covering the costs of services)
- Innovation for acceleration (looking toward the future)

## 2.3 Epidemiology of HIV

To be effective, the global or local response to HIV ought to be evidence-informed. That is why the epidemiology of HIV has been cardinal to the global response since the 1980s. Among others, epidemiology informs which response strategy (whether you are preventing, controlling, eliminating, or eradicating) is to be applied where, when, and how. These concepts are explained in Chap. 1.

De Cock and Jaffe described the epidemiology of the HIV/AIDS epidemic as evolving and highlighted prevention interventions and other factors potentially affecting transmission and spread [9]. Thus, following its recognition in 1981, the HIV/AIDS epidemic has evolved to become one of the greatest challenges in global health [9], having claimed about 36.3 million as of 2020 [8]. There is no vaccine nor cure for HIV as yet. However, increasing access to effective HIV prevention, diagnosis, treatment, and care, including for opportunistic infections, has transformed HIV into a manageable chronic health condition. At the end of 2020, there were an estimated 37.7 million people living with HIV, over two thirds of whom (25.4 million) are in the WHO African Region. Nine countries in Southern Africa account for less than 2% of the world's population, but now they represent about one third of global HIV infections [9]. In 2020, 680,000 people died from HIV-related causes, and 1.5 million people acquired HIV. Recently, Govender et al. analyzed rates and trends for prevalence, incidence, mortality, and disability adjusted life years in different regions of the world. Forecasting was used to estimate disease burden up to 2040 [10]. Although many countries have witnessed a decrease in the incidence, for Russia, Ukraine, Portugal, Brazil, Spain, and the United States, the rates of new cases are rising since 2010. Mortality rates are falling globally, currently at 11 deaths per 100,000 population, forecast to decrease to 8.5 deaths by 2040 [10]. Prevalence continues to increase, with South Africa, Nigeria, Mozambique, India, Kenya, and the United States having the highest burden. The total number as well as the rates of new HIV infections are rising every year in Europe, South America, North America, and other regions over the last decade – contributing to the world's collective failure to meeting the 90-90-90 targets in 2020 and putting the 90-90-90 targets (to be achieved by 2030) and the 95-95-95 targets (also to be achieved by 2030) in jeopardy [10]. Described earlier, the UNAIDS 2020 targets of 90-90-90 aimed to get 90% of people living with HIV (PLHIV) diagnosed, 90% of those diagnosed on treatment, and 90% of those on treatment virally suppressed. The 2030 targets aim at attaining a 90% reduction in new HIV infection, 90% reduction in stigma and discrimination, and 90% reduction in AIDS-related deaths, while the newly proposed 95-95-95 aim to improve on the 2020 targets.

The greatest challenge in terms of prevention has been in the global community of men who have sex with men (MSM) in which HIV remains endemic at high prevalence. The most promising interventions include male circumcision and use of ART to reduce infectiousness. Preventive measures such as condom use, prevention of mother-to-child transmission, voluntary male medical circumcision, and community awareness campaigns have been less successful than anticipated perhaps due to unaddressed systems issues [11]. Antiretroviral therapy had more PLHIV, and thus it was anticipated that the incidence and mortality will decrease. Pre-exposure prophylaxis (PrEP), ART leading to viral suppression made the theoretical construct of "Undetectable = Untransmittable" (U = U) a reality, and PMTCT for MTCT has been adjudged one of the most potent HIV interventions available [12, 13]. HIV infections vary by regions, even within countries [14, 15]. These variations in HIV prevalence have important implications in the efforts to bring HIV pandemic under control.

## 2.4  HIV Surveillance and Testing/Screening

Outlined in Chap. 1, surveillance is the ongoing systematic collection, analysis, and interpretation of data and the timely dissemination of these data to those who need them [16]. In the public health, aside from surveillance, "testing," "screening," and "case finding" are relevant tools. Testing is the application of a test or measurement to selected individuals for the purpose of identifying a disease or medical condition. The individuals might be selected for testing because there is a clinical reason or risk factors that suggest the presence of the condition. Screening generally refers to the application of a test to all individuals in a defined population. Screening is commonly instituted for the purpose of case finding-identifying a previously unknown or unrecognized condition in apparently healthy or asymptomatic persons and offering pre-symptomatic "treatment" to those so identified. Screening is also sometimes done for surveillance purposes: to monitor the incidence or prevalence of a disease in a defined population over time or to compare the incidence or prevalence among different populations [17].

Other public health practices used to protect the public by preventing exposure to people who have or may have a contagious disease are isolation and quarantine. Isolation separates sick people with a contagious disease from people who are not sick. Quarantine separates and restricts the movement of people who were or may have been exposed to a contagious disease. These people may have been exposed to a disease and do not know it, or they may have the disease but do not show symptoms.

This aspect of public health practice, "surveillance" was resorted to during the early days of HIV. For surveillance to be effective, there must be a case definition of the condition under surveillance. In 1982, the US Centers for Disease Control and Prevention (CDC) published its first case definition for AIDS as "a disease at least moderately predictive of a defect in cell-mediated immunity, occurring in a person with no known case for diminished resistance to that disease. Such diseases include Kaposi's sarcoma, pneumocystis carinii pneumonia and serious opportunistic infections" [18]. Having a case definition for this emerging disease at that time set the stage for disease surveillance which focused on the number of individuals diagnosed with AIDS. This meant that cases were reported only after the virus had inflicted harm on the host to the extent that AIDS was manifested [19]. It was estimated during the time that the incubation period – from HIV infection to frank manifestation of AIDS – was approximately 10 years.

Benefiting from hindsight, experts note that the surveillance system then was only able to track where the epidemic had been instead of where it was heading. The surveillance system had to be restructured to include focusing on incidence of HIV infections to appropriately guide prevention planning, resource allocation, and evaluation of interventions at all levels. The identification of the causative agent led the CDC to revise its case definition in 1985 to reflect that AIDS is caused by a newly identified virus. HIV case reporting was then introduced as a surveillance tool in several national HIV/AIDS surveillance systems, in addition to AIDS case reporting and sentinel HIV sero-surveillance. Restructuring of the surveillance system was timely as antiretroviral drugs became available and provided long-term survival among infected persons and a slow progression to AIDS, thereby making AIDS prevalence a less reliable marker of the evolving epidemic. Developing countries on the other hand had to apply a case definition of AIDS based on clinical criteria as a result of lack of resources and technical capacity. Tuberculosis, herpes zoster, and some sexually transmitted diseases were identified as markers for vulnerability of populations to HIV; hence, surveillance systems were tuned to identify such populations and direct interventions to them. Surveillance systems also make use of data collected from voluntary testing and counselling, testing for diagnostic purposes, or the screening of donated blood [20].

## 2.5   HIV Testing

HIV testing and counselling (HTC) is an important entry point for a range of services including HIV testing, prevention, management, prevention of mother-to-child transmission (PMTCT), and other support services. Extending HIV testing beyond blood donors required extra caution, and emphasis was placed on voluntarism. Voluntary counseling and testing (VCT) was hence adopted. It consists of three key components which include pre- and post-test counselling, informed written consent, and confidentiality. Later, reports on the survival benefit of ART sparked a new discussion among public health professionals about incorporating HIV testing and treatment in standard clinical practice in settings where ART was available. Also, epidemiologic studies showed that very few of people with the infected knew of their status, with most of them becoming aware at the end stage of the disease. To boost the uptake of HIV testing and other services, provider-initiated HIV testing and counselling was introduced to be practiced in healthcare settings where healthcare providers assume consent unless patients opt not to have the test done [21]. In 2015, the WHO in consultation with stakeholders adopted "HIV testing services" (HTS) in place of HIV testing and counselling to encompass the full range of services that should be provided together with HIV testing and counselling, including linkage to appropriate HIV prevention and treatment care services and other clinical and support services. They also recommended supporting HTS with trained lay providers and the potential of HIV self-testing to increase access and coverage of HIV testing as part of strategies toward achieving near universal testing targets [22].

Contact tracing and linkage to care at the time when no effective treatment was available, coupled with ethical issues surrounding privacy and confidentiality of HIV tests, were not common. HIV case reporting data did not include infected individuals who had not tested as well as those who used anonymous testing sites, making the data unrepresentative of the larger population of infected persons [23]. In recent times, sentinel surveillance, a method of collecting incidence or prevalence data from targeted samples of certain populations is used as a proxy to estimate the incidence in the population as a whole [24]. Sentinel surveillance of pregnant women seeking antenatal care in public health facilities has and is being used in some countries to estimate HIV prevalence [25]. This is supplemented by surveillance in high-risk individuals attending specialist clinics for STIs and national population-based household surveys [26]. An effective HIV surveillance system enables directing of prevention strategies to at-risk groups and monitoring the course of the epidemic [26]. Largely the HIV statistics/HIV numbers (HIV incidence, HIV prevalence, AIDS incidence, AIDS prevalence, reported cases, official cases, estimated cases, actual cases) that are used to inform programming are generated through surveillance, data collected during routine service provision, and other processes.

Regarding AIDS statistics, some of the frequent questions have been what do these numbers mean? And how are the numbers generated? The frequent response has been that they are generating through counting or estimations and sometimes guestimations. In epidemiology – a branch of public health, we count. We count from nuptiality (marriages) through natality (births), to deaths (mortality), and everything in between. With this ageless practice of counting, it is intriguing to be encumbered with controversies about counting HIV or AIDS numbers (e.g., HIV cases, AIDS deaths). I will attempt to throw more light regarding how these numbers are generated. This is relevant if public health practitioners are to be able to address the age-old syndemic of HIV and the infodemia [27] associated with it and other public health challenges. Not only has the pandemic made worst by infodemia; the infodemia is made worst by lay epidemiologists on social media.

Let's take HIV cases (morbidity in this case). These cases represent cases that have been counted or estimated. It is distinct from morbidity rate, which is either the prevalence or incidence of HIV cases, and also from the incidence rate (the number of newly appearing HIV cases of the disease per unit of time). Mortality rate (also HIV death rate) is a measure of the number of AIDS-related deaths in a particular population, taking into consideration the size of that population, at a given time. This may be expressed as crude death rates and standardized death rates. Whether it be crude or standardized rate, one of the most important considerations is the source of the data from which the rates are derived. In most cases there are few if any ways to obtain exact mortality rates (actual counts), so public health professionals would usually estimate or predict these rates. However, due to many challenges (e.g., health infrastructure-related limitations, health resource-related limitations, varying definitional perspectives, and even politics), these rates can be difficult to count, to estimate, to predict, or to guestimate. To illustrate, AIDS deaths may be reported deaths (officially reported deaths by a designated government agency), estimated deaths (derived from government experts/agencies or academics), or actual deaths (deaths that are actually counted or recorded through official registries. Actual deaths or actual counts are the Holy Grail for public health epidemiologists. Aside from deaths, HIV incidence and prevalence are other important numbers. Calculations of HIV incidence (rates) or HIV incident cases are usually as of April 1 of the following calendar year, while HIV prevalence (rates) are computed as of December 31 of the preceding year.

## 2.6  HIV Prevention Strategies: From Classic Public Health Interventions to Modern Innovations

There are three mechanisms involved in the transmission of HIV: sexual contact, exposure to infected blood or blood products, and perinatal or mother-to-child transmission. Sexual transmission is the most predominant mode of transmission worldwide [28]. Aside from the individual biological and behavioral risk factors that influence vulnerability to HIV, economic, socio-cultural, and environmental factors are inevitably involved in determining individual or population vulnerability to HIV infection. Hence, a multi-sectoral approach is required to make prevention interventions successful [29].

Strategies to prevent HIV transmission in the early years mostly focused on "harm reduction" or reduction of individual risk factors among seronegative populations, with little attention paid to structural factors [30]. The male condom was one of the first traditional public health prevention methods to be introduced. It was proven to be cost-effective and effective at reducing the transmission risk of HIV by 95% with consistent and correct use [31, 32].

Condom promotion, distribution, and social marketing programs were introduced in several populations, resulting in a markedly higher use of condoms. The ABC (abstinence, be faithful, and use a condom) approach was used particularly in Africa to change sexual behaviors in at-risk groups. In other parts of the world, behavioral interventions targeted changing risky sexual behaviors among homosexual men, heterosexual men and women, and needle-exchange programs for injection drug users. Behavior change strategies allowed the message or the mode of delivery to be tailored to suit the targeted population in different settings. Soon, STI screening and treatment programs, treatment of substance abuse, and mental disorders were added to the growing arsenal of preventive strategies [29]. The WHO in 2007 recommended the use of voluntary male medical circumcision (VMMC) for men, after it was found to provide lifelong risk reduction of 60% from female-to-male HIV transmission [33]. Following the recommendation, VMMC programs were rolled out in several populations where male circumcision was not a common practice [34].

It is understood that no single intervention on its own is sufficient to stop the epidemic. Curbing HIV/AIDS epidemic requires a context-based approach, bearing in mind the stigma, economic factors, and social and gender norms that may prevail in different settings [29]. Combination prevention was introduced to remedy the weaknesses of previous HIV prevention strategies. Prevention programs had to be tailored to national and local contexts, using a mix of biomedical, behavioral, and structural interventions aimed at addressing immediate risks and underlying vulnerability, thoughtfully planned and managed on multiple levels to attain sustained reductions in HIV incidence in diverse settings [30]. This feat cannot be attained without a thorough understanding of the stage and nature of the HIV epidemic in a particular setting, referred to as "know your epidemic, know your response" [35], which requires an understanding of the virus, individual experiences and the socio-environmental determinants, and the continuous shifting of social connections and practices that have shared or different meanings to people involved [36]. From the foregoing, HIV prevention strategies/intervention have truly evolved. The overview includes behavior change interventions, biomedical strategies, social justice and human rights, and treatment/antiretroviral/STI treatments. Leadership and scaling up of treatment and prevention efforts but also community involvement are critical. These are examined in depth in Chap. 3.

## 2.7   Recent Innovations in HIV Prevention

The triple-combination therapy when adhered to does not only prolong survival for infected individuals but has a positive effect in a population where the use of ART is widespread, both among seropositive persons as care and among seronegative persons (with an increased risk of infection) as prophylaxis. This creates a prevention-care synergy, where individual and community viral suppression is achieved, thereby greatly reducing the incidence of HIV infections [29]. Treatment as prevention (TasP) is a modern innovation in HIV prevention that has shown a lot of promise in the control of the epidemic and, when implemented effectively, can reduce transmissibility by 96% [37, 38]. With TasP, the UNAIDS had the motivation to surmise that elimination of the epidemic is possible by year 2030, if countries are able to have 90% of HIV-infected persons tested, 90% of those with knowledge of their HIV-positive serostatus on ART, and 90% of those on ART virally suppressed; thus, the United Nations General Assembly set the 90-90-90 fast-tract targets for year 2020, toward ending the epidemic in 2030 [39]. TasP can be applied in two ways: scale-up of ART uptake among infected persons to attain individual and community viral suppression and the use of ART as pre-exposure prophylaxis (PrEP) to prevent HIV infections among people at high risk of getting infected [34]. For HIV-infected persons, the aim is to reduce the transmission of HIV by testing and identifying people with the infection and initiating treatment regardless of medical eligibility [40]. TasP is as effective as testing and early identification, linkage to care, retention in care, adherence, and viral load suppression. PrEP on the other hand consists of antiretroviral medications that are taken by HIV-negative people before potential exposure to HIV in order to reduce the risk of transmission. The risk of HIV is even lowered if PrEP is used in combination with other preventive methods like condoms. The WHO guidelines recommend PrEP for people who are at a substantial risk of HIV infection such as sex workers, MSM, injection drug users, people with HIV-infected partners, and people (especially women) who are unable to negotiate condom use or control sexual encounters as a result of socio-cultural barriers [41].

## 2.8 Prevention of Mother-to-Child Transmission of HIV (PMTCT)

HIV-positive mothers can transmit the virus to their children during pregnancy, childbirth, and through breastfeeding (this is also known as vertical transmission). The estimated risk of mother-to-child transmission (MTCT) without any intervention from the period of pregnancy to 18 to 24 months of breastfeeding is between 30 and 45%. PMTCT programs have spearheaded HIV care and treatment innovations and have prevented about 1.4 million new infections among children between 2010 and 2018 worldwide [42].

The WHO recommendations for PMTCT have been through a few revisions. In 2015 the WHO published recommendations requiring all pregnant and breastfeeding women living with HIV to be given lifelong treatment regardless of CD4 count. This is known as Option B+, and it set the stage for the "Treat All" policy which ended all the WHO clinical staging and CD4 thresholds previously used to determine ART eligibility. All persons diagnosed with HIV should be offered ART immediately. To prevent MTCT, a comprehensive four-pronged approach is adopted. They include:

- Primary prevention of HIV among women of reproductive age (15–49 years).
- Prevention of unintended pregnancies in women living with HIV.
- Prevention of HIV transmission from a woman living with HIV to her baby (includes use of ARV, safe obstetric practices, and safe infant feeding). ART in this context is given as treatment for the mother and prophylaxis for the child during the pre-natal and post-natal periods.
- Providing long-term follow-up of mother-infant pair and their families [41].

The rapid scale-up of Option B+ in several countries resulted in increased enrollment and a reduction in new infections. Elimination of MTCT has been achieved in Armenia, Belarus, the Caribbean, Cuba, and Thailand, whereas Ethiopia, South Africa, and Tanzania have MTCT rates below 5%, moving toward elimination [43]. Several other countries especially in sub-Saharan Africa have some catching up to do. Globally, about 90% of new infections in children below 15 years are due to MTCT [44]. Action must be taken to develop strategies to get other countries on track to elimination by building on the successes achieved so far [45]. In Ghana, national HIV prevention strategic guidelines take aim at virtual elimination of mother-to-child transmission (eMTCT) of HIV, as well as sustaining and scaling up ART. Elimination in this context refers to MTCT rate of less than 5% at 12 months of age among children born to HIV-positive mothers in breastfeeding populations or MTCT rate less than 2% at 6 weeks of age among children born to HIV-positive mothers in formula feeding settings and a 90% reduction in new pediatric HIV infections.

As outlined above, infant feeding interventions has been a major component of PMTCT. Prior to the emergency of HIV, breastfeeding had been known to be the gold standard for infant feeding, and it was the number one recommendation a health worker would give to a mother on her feeding option. There was no doubt about its benefits to both the mother and child until HIV was found to be in breast-milk in 1985. This discovery created a chasm in the scientific community between those who for fear of transmission of the virus recommend replacement feeding because it carries zero risk for post-natal MTCT and those who for fear of other potential causes of infant morbidity and mortality do not recommend replacement feeding in some contexts. The WHO and other UN agencies responded to this contention with consensus declarations which metamorphosed HIV and infant feeding guidelines or recommendations. These recommendations have had their fair share of revisions. For HIV-negative women and women with unknown status, breastfeeding remains the gold standard; infants should be breastfed exclusively for the first 6 months of life, thereafter receiving nutritionally adequate and safe complementary foods, while breastfeeding continues up to 24 months or beyond. The WHO in 2010 recommended replacement feeding for HIV-positive women and their HIV-exposed infants only when it met certain criteria known as AFASS – acceptability, feasibility, affordability, sustainability, and safety – as is generally perceived to be in the developed world. If replacement feeding cannot fulfill the AFASS criteria, exclusive breastfeeding is recommended during the first 6 months of life with antepartum and post-natal ARV prophylaxis or treatments given where available. Although this recommendation seems reasonable and appropriate, it raises concerns on infant feeding modalities and the impact it can have on mothers in breastfeeding populations or resource-limited settings. Choosing any of the two options for a woman in such contexts presents unique challenges that may undermine efforts to reduce MTCT. Firstly, research has revealed that choosing replacement feeding is tantamount to announcing your HIV status and is accompanied by the stigma and discrimination. Other barriers to replacement feeding include high costs of replacement foods and fuel for cooking, unreliable supple of electrical power, poor access to safe water, and storage facilities. On the other hand, choosing the other option of exclusive breastfeeding, the mother faces social pressures (since relatives and neighbors are part of the decision-making team surrounding infant feeding) to practice mixed feeding and water supplementation which increases the risk of childhood morbidities and mortalities. Exclusive breastfeeding and exclusive replacement feedings are perceived to be culturally and socially unacceptable [46, 47].

Overall, the global response to HIV has made enormous gains, but challenges remain. HIV remains a global public health threat with about 37 million people living with the virus worldwide, and sub-Saharan Africa continues to bear the highest burden. Millions of people living with HIV or at risk of contracting HIV do not have access to treatment and prevention services. There is still no cure or a vaccine for the virus. There is a need to incorporate the abounding social challenges to mount an effective and efficient attack against the epidemic. The road to ending the AIDS epidemic still seems far; however, persistence and relentlessness are sure to take us to our desired destination. That said, no public health response to HIV will chalk a truly durable and sustainable success without addressing – alongside the medical challenges and social challenges associated with HIV – such as stigma, discrimination, access to services, AIDS denialism, misinformation, and conspiracy theories but also new and disinformation and AIDS infodemia

# References

 1. Koop CE. The early days of AIDS, as i remember them. In: Annals of the forum for collaborative HIV research: 2011; 2011.
 2. Quinn TC. AIDS in Africa: a retrospective. Bull World Health Organ. 2001;79(12):1156–67.
 3. CDC. Principles of epidemiology in public health practice, third edition: an introduction to applied epidemiology and biostatistics. Available at https://www.cdcgov/csels/dsepd/ss1978/lesson1/section11html. 2012.
 4. WHO. International health regulations and emergency committees Available at https://www.whoint/news-room/q-a-detail/what-are-the-international-health-regulations-and-emergency-committees. 2019.
 5. Rosenwald MS. History's deadliest pandemics, from ancient Rome to modern America. Washington Post. https://www.washingtonpostcom/graphics/2020/local/retropolis/coronavirus-deadliest-pandemics/. 2021.
 6. Merson MH. The HIV–AIDS pandemic at 25 – the global response. N Engl J Med. 2006;354(23):2414–7.
 7. WHO. WHO declares a global health emergency. Retrieved from https://www.aidsmapcom/news/oct-2003/who-declares-global-health-emergency. 2003.
 8. WHO. HIV/ADIS factsheet. https://www.whoint/news-room/fact-sheets/detail/hiv-aids. 2021.
 9. De Cock KM, Jaffe HW, Curran JW. The evolving epidemiology of HIV/AIDS. AIDS. 2012;26(10):1205–13.
10. Govender RD, Hashim MJ. Global epidemiology of HIV/AIDS: a resurgence in North America and Europe. 2021;11(3):296–301.
11. Kumar A, Singh B, Kusuma YS. Counselling services in prevention of mother-to-child transmission (PMTCT) in Delhi, India: an assessment through a modified version of UNICEF-PPTCT tool. J Epidemiol Glob Health. 2015;5(1):3–13.
12. Maemun S, Mariana N, Rusli A, Mahkota R, Purnama TB. Early initiation of ARV therapy among TB-HIV patients in Indonesia prolongs survival rates! J Epidemiol Glob Health. 2020;10(2):164–7.
13. Nguyen VK, Greenwald ZR, Trottier H, Cadieux M, Goyette A, Beauchemin M, Charest L, Longpré D, Lavoie S, Tossa HG, et al. Incidence of sexually transmitted infections before and after preexposure prophylaxis for HIV. AIDS. 2018;32(4):523–30.

14. Elgalib A, Shah S, Al-Wahaibi A, Al-Habsi Z, Al-Fouri M, Lau R, Al-Kindi H, Al-Rawahi B, Al-Abri S. The epidemiology of HIV in Oman, 1984-2018: a nationwide study from the middle east. J Epidemiol Glob Health. 2020;10(3):222–9.
15. Memish ZA, Al-Tawfiq JA, Filemban SM, Qutb S, Fodail A, Ali B, Darweeish M. Antiretroviral therapy, CD4, viral load, and disease stage in HIV patients in Saudi Arabia: a 2001-2013 cross-sectional study. J Infect Dev Cries. 2015;9(7):765–9.
16. Thacker SB, Berkelman RL. Public health surveillance in the United States. Epidemiol Rev. 1988;10:164–90.
17. IOM, Institute of Medicine (US) Committee on Perinatal Transmission of HIV, National Research Council (US) and Institute of Medicine (US) Board on Children, Youth, and Families, Stoto MA, Almario DA, McCormick MC, editors. Reducing the odds: preventing perinatal transmission of HIV in the United States. Washington (DC): National Academies Press (US); 1999. 2, Public Health Screening Programs. Available from: https://www.ncbi.nlm.nih.gov/books/NBK230552/. 1999.
18. Control CFD. Acquired immunodeficiency syndrome, AIDS: recommendations and guidelines, November 1982-December 1987: Centers for Disease Control, Public Health Service, Department of Health and …; 1988.
19. Gostin LO, Ward JW, Baker AC. National HIV case reporting for the United States. A defining moment in the history of the epidemic. N Engl J Med. 1997;337(16):1162–7.
20. Riedner G, Dehne KL. HIV/AIDS surveillance in developing countries: experiences and issues: Deutsche Gesellschaft für Technische Zusammenarbeit. 1999.
21. Baggaley R, Hensen B, Ajose O, Grabbe KL, Wong VJ, Schilsky A, Lo YR, Lule F, Granich R, Hargreaves J. From caution to urgency: the evolution of HIV testing and counselling in Africa. Bull World Health Organ. 2012;90(9):652–658b.
22. WHO. Consolidated Guidelines on HIV Testing Services. 2015.
23. Stoto M. Public health surveillance: a historical review with a focus on HIV/AIDS. Santa Monica: RAND Health: DRU-3074-IOM. Available from: https://www.rand.org/pubs/drafts/2005/DRU3074.pdf. 2003.
24. Johri M, Kaplan EH, Levi J, Novick A. New approaches to HIV surveillance: means and ends. Summary report of conference held at Yale University, 21-22 May 1998, by the Law, Policy and Ethics Core, Center for Interdisciplinary Research on AIDS, Yale University. AIDS Public Policy J. 1999;14(4):136–46.
25. Buthelezi UE, Davidson CL, Kharsany ABM. Strengthening HIV surveillance: measurements to track the epidemic in real time. Afr J AIDS Res. 2016;15(2):89–98.
26. Ruiz MS, Gable AR, Kaplan EH, Stoto MA, Fineberg HV, Trussell J. No time to lose: getting more from HIV prevention. Washington (DC): National Academies Press; 2001.
27. Zarocostas J. How to fight an infodemic. Lancet. 2020;395(10225):676.
28. Askew I, Berer M. The contribution of sexual and reproductive health services to the fight against HIV/AIDS: a review. Reprod Health Matters. 2003;11(22):51–73.
29. Bertozzi S, Padian NS, Wegbreit J, DeMaria LM, Feldman B, Gayle H, Gold J, Grant R, Isbell MT. HIV/AIDS prevention and treatment. In: Jamison DT, Breman JG, Measham AR, Alleyne G, Claeson M, Evans DB, Jha P, Mills A, Musgrove P, editors. Disease control priorities in developing countries. Washington, DC/New York: The International Bank for Reconstruction and Development/The World Bank Oxford University Press; 2006.
30. UNAIDS. Combination HIV prevention: tailoring and coordinating biomedical, behavioural and structural strategies to reduce new HIV infections. Available at https://www.unaidsorg/en/resources/documents/2010/20101006_JC2007_Combination_Prevention_paper. 2010.
31. Anderson JE. Condom use and HIV risk among US adults. Am J Public Health. 2003;93(6):912–4.
32. Grangeiro A, Ferraz D, Calazans G, Zucchi EM, Díaz-Bermúdez XP. The effect of prevention methods on reducing sexual risk for HIV and their potential impact on a large-scale: a literature review. Revista Brasileira de Epidemiologia. 2015;18:43–62.

33. PEPFAR. 2019 Annual report to Congress. Retrieved from https://www.stategov/wp-content/uploads/2019/09/PEPFAR2019ARCpdf. 2019.
34. McCarten-Gibbs M, Allinder S. The evolution and future of HIV prevention technology: an HIV policy primer. 2019.
35. UNAIDS. Practical guidelines for intensifying HIV prevention. 2007.
36. Stephenson N. A social public health. Am J Public Health. 2011;101(7):1159.
37. Cohen MS, Chen YQ, McCauley M, Gamble T, Hosseinipour MC, Kumarasamy N, Hakim JG, Kumwenda J, Grinsztejn B, Pilotto JH, et al. Prevention of HIV-1 infection with early antiretroviral therapy. N Engl J Med. 2011;365(6):493–505.
38. Cremin I, Alsallaq R, Dybul M, Piot P, Garnett G, Hallett TB. The new role of antiretrovirals in combination HIV prevention: a mathematical modelling analysis. AIDS. 2013;27(3):447–58.
39. UNAIDS. Fast-Track – ending the AIDS epidemic by 2030 I UNAIDS. Retrieved July 11, 2021, from https://www.unaidsorg/en/resources/documents/2014/JC2686_WAD2014report. 2014.
40. Diethelm P, McKee M. Denialism: what is it and how should scientists respond? Eur J Public Health. 2009;19(1):2–4.
41. WHO. WHO expands recommendation on oral pre-exposure prophylaxis of HIV infection (PrEP). 2015.
42. UNAIDS. Miles to go: global AIDS update. 2018.
43. UNAIDS. UNAIDS AIDSinfo. Retrieved from https://www.aidsinfounaidsorg/. 2017.
44. Ciaranello AL, Perez F, Keatinge J, Park JE, Engelsmann B, Maruva M, Walensky RP, Dabis F, Chu J, Rusibamayila A, et al. What will it take to eliminate pediatric HIV? Reaching WHO target rates of mother-to-child HIV transmission in Zimbabwe: a model-based analysis. PLoS Med. 2012;9(1):e1001156.
45. Vrazo AC, Sullivan D, Ryan Phelps B. Eliminating mother-to-child transmission of HIV by 2030: 5 strategies to ensure continued progress. Glob Health Sci Pract. 2018;6(2):249–56.
46. Laar AK, Amankwa B, Asiedu C. Prevention-of-mother-to-child-transmission of HIV services in Sub-Saharan Africa: a qualitative analysis of healthcare providers and clients challenges in Ghana. Int J MCH AIDS. 2014;2(2):244–9.
47. Laar A, Ampofo W, Tuakli J, Quakyi I. Infant feeding choices and experiences of HIV-positive mothers from two Ghanaian districts. J AIDS HIV Res. 2009;1(2):23–33.

# Chapter 3
# HIV Interventions: Which Should Count? Which Should Not? And Why Not?

## 3.1 Introduction

Since its emergence in the 1980s, the scientific community has provided evidence to support the claim that the causative agent of acquired immunodeficiency syndrome (AIDS) is human immunodeficiency virus (HIV) [1]. HIV causes AIDS by undermining the immune system, eventually resulting in death [1]. HIV has since been isolated and photographed and its genome fully described [2]. Although no cure or vaccine has yet been discovered, scientific advances have resulted in the development of countermeasures including AIDS medications both for therapeutic and preventative prophylactic uses. An array of successful interventions exists. For instance, the global public health literature is replete with success stories of prevention of mother-to-child transmission (PMTCT) of HIV and the clinical and public health benefits of antiretroviral medications (ARVs) [3]. There remain important challenges, nevertheless. Concerns relating to equity in AIDS response measures reign. Although equity is not an intervention [4], AIDS interventions are characterized by increasing inequity. Few will debate the claim that equity is not the primary goal driving core AIDS policies and programs. Indeed, equity is often consciously and easily sacrificed for other goals. To this effect, some commentators have quizzed whether it is reasonable to expect that interventions generated from systems that perpetuate inequities to lead to equity. Hay [4] suggests that it is reasonable, but only if intentional disruptions are injected to perturb the iniquitous equilibrium. This chapter pays heed.

With no cure or vaccine currently, HIV and AIDS countermeasures are heavily skewed toward prevention and rightly so. The question, however, is the nature, scope, depth, and breadth of those preventative interventions. HIV prevention programs are generically conceptualized as interventions that aim to halt its transmission. After years of research, advocacy, and policy initiatives, such programs currently include preventing the transmission of HIV through a complementary

© The Author(s), under exclusive license to Springer Nature Switzerland AG 2022
A. Laar, *Balancing the Socio-political and Medico-ethical Dimensions of HIV*,
SpringerBriefs in Public Health, https://doi.org/10.1007/978-3-031-09191-9_3

combination of behavioral, biomedical, and structural strategies. These countermeasures are implemented to either protect an individual and their community or are rolled out as public health policies which seek the same goal [5].

Either for political expediency or lack of scientific evidence, HIV prevention programs in the beginning (the 1980s–1990s) focused primarily on preventing the sexual transmission of HIV through behavior change. For a number of years, the "*a*bstinence, *b*e faithful, and *c*ondom use" – code-named the ABC approach – was the mainstay of HIV epidemic control measures in many regions of the world. By the mid-2000s, it became evident that effective HIV prevention needed to take into account underlying socio-cultural, economic, political, legal, and other contextual factors [6]. Thus, as the complex nature of the global HIV epidemic became clear, other forms of countermeasures were brought onboard. Science won! But politics did not fissile out of HIV "science," HIV programming, or HIV policy-making. ABC-type HIV interventions remained and were vertically deployed in some settings – for a long time. They still do albeit in limited settings.

Over time, the scientific community and lay policy-makers learned that, to a considerable extent, the countermeasures that are multilayered are relatively more efficacious and yield the desired dividend. For example, the global decline in new HIV infections nearly 25 years since the advent of antiretroviral medications (ARVs) was attributed to the effective layering of these interventions. The UNAIDS reported a decline by 16% between 2010 and 2018. In epidemiologic framing, HIV may thus be said to have been controlled, and there are now musings of HIV elimination in some jurisdictions [7]. In Chap. 1, I discussed the epidemiologic concepts of the level of disease and hierarchy of public health interventions. The global public health responses mounted since the founding of the World Health Organization (WHO) have had diseases (also public health events/challenges), prevented, controlled (e.g., malaria), eliminated (e.g., measles), and eradicated (smallpox). The world is yet to record the first case of disease extinction. The seminal work by the US Centers for Disease Control and Prevention (CDC) and Dowdle and Hopkins provides elucidation to these concepts [8, 9]:

- *Disease prevention*: the specific, population-based and individual-based interventions for preventing the occurrence of a disease/health problem (primary prevention), early detection (secondary prevention), and treatment to prevent complications (tertiary prevention). As used here, preventative treatment can include patient education, lifestyle modification, and drugs.
- *Disease control*: reduction of disease incidence, prevalence, morbidity, or mortality to a locally acceptable level as a result of deliberate efforts. Continued intervention measures are required to maintain the reduction. An example is diarrheal diseases.
- *Disease elimination*: reduction to zero of the incidence of a specified infection/disease in a defined geographical area as a result of deliberate efforts. Like control, continued intervention measures are required, e.g., measles and poliomyelitis.

- *Disease eradication*: permanent reduction to zero of the worldwide incidence of infection caused by a specific agent as a result of deliberate efforts; intervention measures are no longer needed. Example: smallpox.
- *Extinction*: the specific infectious agent no longer exists in nature or in the laboratory. Example: none.

Progress in the prevention and control of HIV/AIDS during the last two decades stimulated debate on the possibility of ending HIV/AIDS as a public health threat. Since 2016, UNAIDS and partners have promoted a vision to end HIV/AIDS by 2030 [10]. The third Sustainable Development Goal (SDG-3) has a target to end the epidemic of HIV/AIDS by 2030. Success in regard to the SDG-3 target is defined quantitatively, as a decline in the number of both new HIV infections and "AIDS-related deaths" by 90% between 2010 and 2030 [11]. This resonates with the 90-90-90 fast-track targets that had an end date of 2020 [11]. Referred to many then as an aspirational goal, this aimed to have 90% of PLHIV who know their HIV status, have 90% of people who know their HIV-positive status access treatment, and 90% of people on treatment who achieve sustained viral suppression. Such targets have since been revised to 95-95-95 and to be achieved by 2025. Relevant to this topic is a question asked by Assefa and Gilks [12]. That is the question of what it means to end the epidemic of HIV/AIDS. As outlined above (see hierarchy of public health interventions), public health interventions that aim to "end a public health challenge" can have several scenarios (which include elimination and eradication). In relation to the subject and context under discussion, the problematic fusion of HIV with AIDS responses in the same goal has led to multiple and potentially contradicting targets and slogans [12] – focusing on achieving zero or fewer new HIV cases (HIV incidence), zero or fewer cumulative HIV cases (HIV prevalence), zero or slowed clinical progression to AIDS (AIDS incidence), and zero or fewer deaths in PLHIV (as equivalent to "AIDS-related deaths"). To some experts, ending the epidemic of HIV, in epidemiologic terms, will be achieved when the total number of PLHIV in the country declines to levels only seen at the start of the epidemic [13]. This is possible only when the number of new HIV infections is decreasing to a level that is equal to or less than the number of deaths in PLHIV (irrespective of the cause). However, several regions of the world are lagging on these targets [12]. Other stakeholders advocate for and support a strategy referred to as "epidemic control," which is achieved when the annual number of new HIV infections in a country is less than the number of deaths among PLHIV [14].

Related to epidemic control of HIV or ending HIV/AIDS by 2030 is the concept of virtual elimination of mother-to-child transmission (eMTCT) of HIV defined as reducing the number of vertical transmission of HIV (new child HIV infections) by 90% between 2009 and 2015 or reducing MTCT to <5% [15]. To prevent MTCT, a comprehensive four-pronged approach including (1) primary prevention of HIV infection among women of childbearing age; (2) preventing unintended pregnancies among women living with HIV; (3) preventing HIV transmission from women living with HIV to their infants; and (4) providing appropriate treatment, care, and support to mothers living with HIV and their children and families is recommended

[16]. In countries where breastfeeding is common, the probability of transmission from mother to child without any ARVs was estimated to be about 20–45% (15–25% transmission during pregnancy and 5–20% transmission during breastfeeding) [17]. In resource-rich settings, where all four prongs are well implemented and the most effective ARVs are provided to HIV-positive pregnant women with limited breastfeeding, the level of MTCT has decreased to below 2% [18, 19]. This led to PMTCT being touted as one of the most successful non-vaccine public health intervention since the eradication of smallpox.

That said, HIV appears to be far from being eliminated. In response the UNAIDS in 2017 devised a roadmap and 10-point action plan to help countries meet their targets. Referred to as the Global HIV Prevention Coalition, the roadmap and plan address key issues that are holding back progress – including gaps in political leadership, legal, and policy barriers; gaps in financing prevention; and lack of systematic implementation of combination prevention programs at scale [20]. And yet, in 2020, about 1.3 million adults aged 15 and over who were newly infected with HIV. Current efforts are not leading to a significant enough decline in countries to bring the HIV epidemic to levels low enough to be on track to elimination [21].

## 3.2  HIV Prevention Strategies

Although challenges remain, the HIV prevention programs are working overall – the UNAIDS 2010 Report on the global AIDS epidemic [6] noted. The report indicates that the decline in new HIV infections between 2010 and 2018 was linked with changes in behavior and social norms together with increased knowledge of HIV, and yet two new HIV infections occurred for every individual started on antiretroviral treatment [6]. This called into question the efficiency with which the wide array of existing proven HIV prevention strategies. The report bemoans that prevention efforts as of 2018 have been overwhelmingly focused on reducing individual risk, with fewer efforts made to address structural factors such as socio-cultural, economic, political, legal, and other contextual factors (see Fig. 3.1) [6, 22–24]. To address this documented weaknesses in HIV prevention, the approach known as "combination prevention" and defined as "rights-based, evidence-informed, and community-owned programs that use a mix of biomedical, behavioral, and structural interventions, prioritized to meet the current HIV prevention needs of particular individuals and communities, so as to have the greatest sustained impact on reducing new infections" [6] offers the best prospects. Combination prevention relies on the evidence-informed, strategic, simultaneous use of complementary behavioral, biomedical, and structural prevention strategies. Combination prevention programs operate on different levels (e.g., individual, relationship, community, societal) to address the specific but diverse needs of the populations at risk of HIV infection. Indeed, knowing what we do now about HIV transmission, a multidisciplinary, multi-stakeholder, multi-actor, multi-sectoral approach is required to make prevention interventions successful [25].

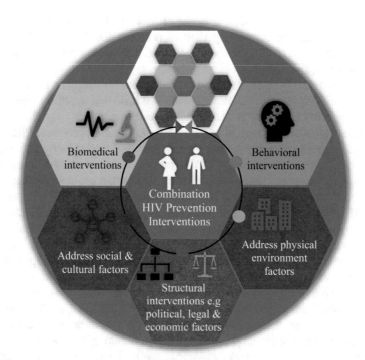

**Fig. 3.1** Effective HIV prevention interventions. (Source: Author's construction based on existing literature [5, 6, 22–24])

Existing evidence and resources including know-how ought to be used efficiently. Options to reduce the risk of acquiring or transmitting HIV are almost numberless. For instance, one can use medicines – antiretroviral medicines as pre-exposure prophylaxis (PrEP), treatment with antiretroviral medicines, voluntary male circumcision (VMMC), behavior change interventions to reduce the number of sexual partners, the use of condoms (male or female), the use of microbicides, etc. Indeed, one can decide to have only low-risk sex or abstinence. All of these can effectively reduce HIV transmission and acquisition risk. As some options are more effective than others, the deployment of combining prevention strategies as noted above is reasonable. On treatment, the use of triple-combination therapy when adhered to does not only prolong survival for infected individuals but has a positive effect in a population where the use of ART is widespread, both among seropositive persons as care and among seronegative persons (with an increases risk of infection) as prophylaxis. This creates a prevention-care synergy, where individual and community viral suppression is achieved, thereby greatly reducing the incidence of HIV infections [25]. Treatment as prevention (TasP) as it's referred to is a modern innovation in HIV prevention that has shown a lot of promise in the control of the epidemic and, when implemented effectively, can reduce transmissibility by 96% [26, 27].

TasP can be applied in two ways: scale-up of ART uptake among infected persons to attain individual and community viral suppression and the use of ART as pre-exposure prophylaxis (PrEP) to prevent HIV infections among people at high risk of getting infected [28].

For HIV-infected persons, the aim is to reduce the transmission of HIV by testing and identifying people with the infection and initiating treatment regardless of medical eligibility [29]. TasP is as effective as testing and early identification, linkage to care, retention in care, adherence, and viral load suppression. PrEP on the other hand consists of antiretroviral medications that are taken by HIV-negative people before potential exposure to HIV in order to reduce the risk of transmission. The risk of HIV is even lowered if PrEP is used in combination with other preventive methods like condoms. The WHO guidelines recommend PrEP for people who are at a substantial risk of HIV infection such as sex workers, MSM, injection drug users, people with HIV-infected partners, and people (especially women) who are unable to negotiate condom use or control sexual encounters as a result of socio-cultural barriers [16]. As outlined, this approach of deploying multiple interventions (some of which have double-duty actions) is referred to as combination prevention. Thus, curbing HIV/AIDS epidemic requires a context-based approach, bearing in mind the stigma, economic factors, and social and gender norms that may prevail in different settings [25]. That is why it's often recommended that the starting point for "combination prevention" programming be evidence synthesis. Through evidence-informed understanding of one's HIV epidemic and the response, sometimes referred to as "know your epidemic, know your response" [30], HIV programmers can make use of the best available research evidence from the biomedical, behavioral, and structural dimensions to plan and execute combination prevention actions.

Both as a concept and in practice, combination prevention advocates for a holistic approach whereby HIV prevention is not a single intervention (such as condom distribution) but the simultaneous use of complementary behavioral, biomedical, social, and structural prevention strategies [6] (also see Figs. 3.2, 3.3, and 3.4). Combination prevention programs consider factors specific to each setting, such as levels of infrastructure, local culture and traditions, as well as populations most affected by HIV. They can be implemented at the individual, community, and population levels [6]. To recognize and address these multivalent needs, combination prevention efforts must meaningfully, sufficiently, and truly recognize the value of the social to the medical. For instance, care and psychosocial support, behavioral interventions, structural interventions, as well as a strong community empowerment must be valued. Efforts that address legal and policy barriers, efforts that strengthen of health and social protection systems, respect for equity, and gender fairness, stigma, and discrimination elimination are extremely important.

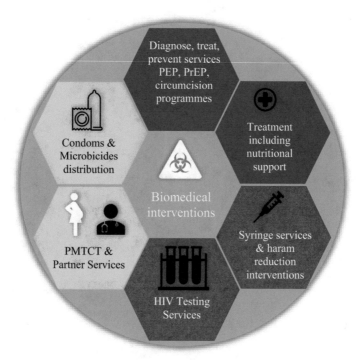

**Fig. 3.2**  Biomedical interventions. (Source: Author's construction based on existing literature [5, 6, 22–24])

## 3.3   Implementing Combination Prevention Programs

Programmatically, combination prevention interventions may deploy biomedical tools to prevent HIV infection both among HIV-negative persons (including the use of male and female condoms, the use of antiretroviral medicines as PrEP, VMMC, behavior change interventions to reduce the number of sexual partners, the use of clean needles and syringes, and getting tested and treated for other STDs) and among those already infected, treatment with ARVs (see TasP) or prevention of HIV superinfection where HIV-positive individuals adopt positive preventive behavior change to avoid contracting another type of the virus (see Fig. 3.2). Of note, biomedical interventions use a mix of clinical and medical approaches to reduce HIV transmission. In order to be effective, biomedical interventions are rarely implemented independently and are often used in conjunction with behavioral interventions [5]. For example, when a man is circumcised, he will often be tested for HIV and receive counselling and education about condom use and safer sex.

Thus, combination prevention recognizes social and behavioral interventions that aim to reduce the risk of HIV transmission by addressing risky behaviors (Fig. 3.3). As such, behavior change communication forms a basic component of

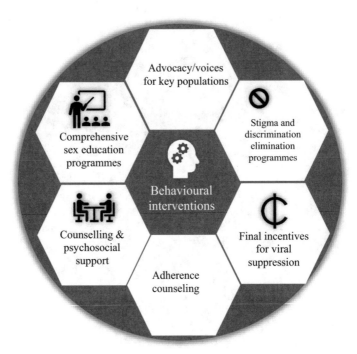

**Fig. 3.3** Behavioral interventions. (Source: Author's construction based on existing literature [5, 6, 22–24])

combination prevention. Interventions in this category include information provision (such as sex education), counselling and other forms of psychosocial support, safe infant feeding guidelines, stigma, and discrimination reduction programs. Effective behavior interventions address the cultural contexts within which risk behaviors occur and aim to stimulate the uptake of HIV prevention services. These programs often feature intensive approaches involving a combination of activities to address multiple outcomes, including knowledge, risk perception, norms, skills, behaviors, and HIV service demand. A behavioral intervention may aim to reduce the number of sexual partners that individuals have, improve treatment adherence among people living with HIV, increase the use of clean needles among people who inject drugs, or increase the consistent and correct use of condoms [5].

Like biomedical interventions, behavioral interventions have limitations. Delivered alone, behavioral interventions are not able to address structural determinants of HIV risk, acquisition, transmission, and treatment prognosis. A renewed public health must address social, cultural, and economic differentials that deny the public the enjoyment of their basic rights. It must also promote justice (politically, economically, socially, and culturally). It must address what Giles-Vernick bemoans is long overdue – meaningful response to the social determinants of health [31] as well as what West and Marteau referred to as "commercial determinants of health" (factors that influence health which stem from the profit motive) and what Gostin

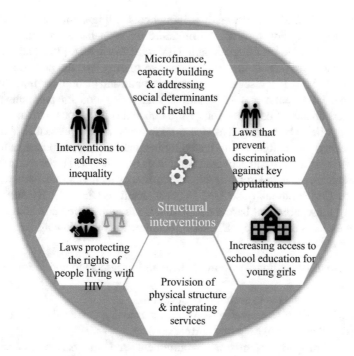

**Fig. 3.4** Structural interventions. (Source: Author's construction based on existing literature [5, 6, 22–24])

et al. termed "legal determinants of health" [32, 33]. They articulate the crucial role of law in achieving global public health through legal instruments, legal capacities, and institutional reforms, as well as a firm commitment to the rule of law.

Termed structural violence, and defined as violence wherein social structures or social institutions harm people by preventing them from meeting their basic needs, Johan Galtung lists examples to include institutionalized adultism, ageism, classism, elitism, ethnocentrism, nationalism, speciesism, racism, and sexism [34]. Neither biomedical nor behavioral interventions are sensitive to these. Paul Farmer links structural violence to social injustice [35], while Wadhwa extends that to include ineffective, inappropriate policy stances as tantamount to structural violence [36]. Addressing structural determinants of HIV risk, acquisition, transmission, and treatment prognosis would require cultural and structural competence and definitely structural interventions.

Structural interventions seek to address underlying factors that make individuals or groups vulnerable to HIV infection. These can be social, economic, political, or environmental. For many people, the simple fact that 90% of the world's HIV infections occur in developing countries is evidence that social, economic, and political structures drive risk behaviors and shape vulnerability [35]. Contrary to theories that poverty acts as an underlying driver of HIV infection in sub-Saharan Africa (SSA), an increasing body of evidence at the national and individual levels indicates that wealthier countries, and wealthier individuals within countries, are at heightened risk for HIV. Fox reviews the literature on what has increasingly become known as the positive-wealth gradient in HIV infection in SSA [36]. The concept of positive-wealth gradient is the counterintuitive finding that the poor do not have higher rates of HIV. Fox discusses the programmatic and theoretical implications of the positive HIV-wealth gradient for traditional behavioral interventions and the social determinants of health literature and concludes by proposing that economic and social policies be leveraged as structural interventions to prevent HIV in SSA.

HIV-related vulnerabilities are fueled by inequalities and prejudices entrenched within the legal, social, and economic structures of society [37]. For example, laws that criminalize same-sex relationships often hinder men who have sex with men from accessing condoms (discussed in great detail in Chap. 5). By successfully addressing these structural barriers, individuals are empowered and able to access HIV prevention services [35]. UNAIDS recommends the following key structural interventions:

- "Strengthen legislation, law enforcement and programs to end intimate partner violence.
- Increase girls' access to secondary education.
- Use cash transfers to empower women economically, to keep them in school and to enable them to make healthy partner choices.
- Remove third-party authorization requirements and other barriers to women and young people's access to HIV and sexual and reproductive health services.
- Decriminalize same-sex relationships, cross-dressing, sex work and drug possession and use for personal consumption.
- Bring to scale community empowerment and other programs that have been proven to reduce stigma, discrimination and marginalization" [6].

That said, it ought to be noted that structural interventions are much more difficult to implement because they attempt to deal with deep-rooted socio-economic issues such as poverty, gender inequality, and social marginalization. They can also be reliant on the cooperation of governments to achieve law or policy reforms.

With this background, the questions of which HIV intervention counts, which does not, or should not are answered. All of the interventions (biomedical, behavioral, and structurally) are mutually reinforcing and should count. I have argued throughout this book that what is required is a meaningful intervention mix. An argument which finds grounding in the philosophy of "social public health" [37]. The concept of social public health resonates with today's public health's interest in empowered communities. It recognizes people not only as individuals but also as connected members of groups, networks, and collectives who interact (talk, negotiate, have sex, use drugs, etc.) together. In response to HIV, people and members of communities respond to our programs, in ways that enable them to remain community members – gay, masculine, married, Christian, Muslim, and so on [37]. As discussed in this chapter, the concept of social public health is responsive to both social and structural determinants of health, which Henderson et al. note resonates, to a large extent, with today's public health's interest in empowered communities. It recognizes people not only as individuals but also as connected members of groups, networks, and collectives who interact (talk, negotiate, have sex – whether it be same sex/homosexuals or homosexually experienced heterosexuals, heterosexuals, use drugs, etc.). In response to HIV, people and members of communities respond to public health interventions, in ways that enable them to remain recognized and respected community members – as gay, masculine, married, Christian, Muslim, and so on and so forth.

# References

1. Nowak MA, McMichael AJ. How HIV defeats the immune system. Sci Am. 1995;273(2):58–65.
2. Korber B, Gaschen B, Yusim K, Thakallapally R, Kesmir C, Detours V. Evolutionary and immunological implications of contemporary HIV-1 variation. Br Med Bull. 2001;58:19–42.
3. Dieffenbach CW. Preventing HIV transmission through antiretroviral treatment-mediated virologic suppression: aspects of an emerging scientific agenda. Curr Opin HIV AIDS. 2012;7(2):106–10.
4. Hay K. Equity is not an intervention: implications of evaluation—reflections from India. N Dir Eval. 2017;2017(154):79–89.
5. Avert. HIV prevention programmes overview. Available at https://www.avertorg/professionals/hiv-programming/prevention/overview (2019).
6. UNAIDS. Combination HIV prevention: tailoring and coordinating biomedical, behavioural and structural strategies to reduce new HIV infections. Available at https://www.unaidsorg/en/resources/documents/2010/20101006_JC2007_Combination_Prevention_paper (2010).
7. Nicholas SW. Towards the elimination of pediatric HIV/AIDS in New York State. J Public Health Manag Pract. 2010;16(6):509–11.
8. Dowdle WR, Hopkins DR. The eradication of infectious diseases, vol. 24. New York: NWiley; 1998.
9. CDC P. Recommendations of the international task force for disease eradication. Morb Mortal Wkly Rep. 1993;42:1–38.
10. UNAIDS. United Nations political declaration on ending AIDS sets world on the fast-track to end the epidemic by 2030. New York/Geneva: UNAIDS. http://www.unaidsorg/sites/default/files/20160608_PS_HLM_Political_Declaration_finalpdf (2016).
11. UNAIDS. 90-90-90 An ambitious treatmenttarget to help end the AIDS epidemic. http://www.unaidsorg/sites/default/files/media_asset/90-90-90_en_0pdf (2014).
12. Assefa Y, Gilks CF. Ending the epidemic of HIV/AIDS by 2030: will there be an endgame to HIV, or an endemic HIV requiring an integrated health systems response in many countries? Int J Infect Dis. 2020;100:273–7.
13. Over M. Achieving an AIDS transition: preventing infections to sustain treatment. CGD Books; 2011.
14. PEPFAR. Strategy for accelerating HIV/AIDS epidemic control (2017-2020). 2017. https://www.pepfar.gov/documents/organization/274400pdf. Accessed 7 Nov 2018.
15. Michel S, Tedstrom J. The business of eliminating mother-to-Child HIV transmission. The Huffington Post. 2010.
16. WHO. WHO expands recommendation on oral pre-exposure prophylaxis of HIV infection (PrEP). 2015.
17. De Cock KM, Fowler MG, Mercier E, de Vincenzi I, Saba J, Hoff E, Alnwick DJ, Rogers M, Shaffer N. Prevention of mother-to-child HIV transmission in resource-poor countries: translating research into policy and practice. JAMA. 2000;283(9):1175–82.

18. Townsend CL, Cortina-Borja M, Peckham CS, de Ruiter A, Lyall H, Tookey PA. Low rates of mother-to-child transmission of HIV following effective pregnancy interventions in the United Kingdom and Ireland, 2000-2006. AIDS. 2008;22(8):973–81.
19. European Collaborative Study. The mother-to-child HIV transmission epidemic in Europe: evolving in the East and established in the West. AIDS. 2006;20(10):1419.
20. UNAIDS: Implementation of the HIV prevention 2020 road map: first progress report. 2018.
21. Govender RD, Hashim MJ, Khan MA, Mustafa H, Khan G. Global epidemiology of HIV/AIDS: a resurgence in North America and Europe. J Epidemiol Glob Health. 2021;11(3):296.
22. Division of HIV Prevention, National Center for HIV, Viral Hepatitis, STD, and TB Prevention, Centers for Disease Control and Prevention. Compendium of Evidence-Based Interventions and Best Practices for HIV Prevention Page last reviewed: March 9, 2022.
23. Hankins CA, de Zalduondo BO. Combination prevention: a deeper understanding of effective HIV prevention. AIDS. 2010;24:S70–80.
24. Kurth AE, Celum C, Baeten JM, Vermund SH, Wasserheit JN. Combination HIV prevention: significance, challenges, and opportunities. Curr HIV/AIDS Rep. 2011;8(1):62–72.
25. Bertozzi S, Padian NS, Wegbreit J, DeMaria LM, Feldman B, Gayle H, Gold J, Grant R, Isbell MT. HIV/AIDS prevention and treatment. In: Disease control priorities in developing countries, vol. 2. New York: Oxford University Press; 2006. p. 331–70.
26. Cohen MS, Chen YQ, McCauley M, Gamble T, Hosseinipour MC, Kumarasamy N, Hakim JG, Kumwenda J, Grinsztejn B, Pilotto JH, et al. Prevention of HIV-1 infection with early antiretroviral therapy. N Engl J Med. 2011;365(6):493–505.
27. Cremin I, Alsallaq R, Dybul M, Piot P, Garnett G, Hallett TB. The new role of antiretrovirals in combination HIV prevention: a mathematical modelling analysis. AIDS. 2013;27(3):447–58.
28. McCarten-Gibbs M, Allinder S. The evolution and future of HIV prevention technology: an HIV policy primer. 2019.
29. Diethelm P, McKee M. Denialism: what is it and how should scientists respond? Eur J Pub Health. 2009;19(1):2–4.
30. UNAIDS. Practical guidelines for intensifying HIV prevention. 2007.
31. Giles-Vernick T, Webb JL Jr. Global health in Africa: historical perspectives on disease control. Athens: Ohio University Press; 2013.
32. Gostin LO, Monahan JT, Kaldor J, DeBartolo M, Friedman EA, Gottschalk K, Kim SC, Alwan A, Binagwaho A, Burci GL. The legal determinants of health: harnessing the power of law for global health and sustainable development. Lancet. 2019;393(10183):1857–910.
33. West R, Marteau T. Commentary on Casswell (2013): the commercial determinants of health. Addiction. 2013;108(4):686–7.
34. Galtung J. Violence, peace, and peace research. J Peace Res. 1969;6(3):167–91.
35. Farmer PE, Nizeye B, Stulac S, Keshavjee S. Structural violence and clinical medicine. PLoS Med. 2006;3(10):e449.
36. Wadhwa V. Structural violence and women's vulnerability to HIV/AIDS in India: understanding through a "grief model" framework. Ann Assoc Am Geogr. 2012;102(5):1200–8.
37. Henderson K, Worth H, Aggleton P, Kippax S. Enhancing HIV prevention requires addressing the complex relationship between prevention and treatment. Glob Public Health. 2009;4(2):117–30.

# Chapter 4
# Access to Life-Saving Public Health Goods by Persons Infected with or Affected by HIV

## 4.1 Introduction

Access is an important concept in public health with far-reaching cultural, socio-political, and economic implications. Assuring equitable access to life-saving health commodities remains a challenge globally. Access (to medicine) as conceived by the World Health Organization (WHO) refers to the reasonable ability for people to get medicines required to achieve health. As a right, this first emerged as a social right in [1] and in [2]. Efforts that assure true access to medications provide a crucial entry point for universal health coverage (UHC) and other actions that aim to improve overall health. According to the WHO, UHC is realized when "all people have access to the health services they need, when and where they need them, without financial or other hardships. UHC encompasses the full range of essential health services, from health promotion to prevention, treatment, rehabilitation, and palliative care." Access to affordable, quality primary healthcare is the foundation of UHC, but globally around 3.5 billion people do not receive the health services they need [3]. Another 100 million are pushed into extreme poverty each year because of out-of-pocket spending on health [3]. Aside from availability of medicines, and health professionals who deliver them, other determinants of access to healthcare are socio-cultural, organizational, economic, and geographic in nature but also what John Galtung [4] referred to as structural violence. By this, he meant a form of violence wherein social structures or social institutions harm people by preventing them from meeting their basic needs. Although less visible, it is by far the most lethal form of violence, through causing excess deaths – deaths that would not occur in more equal societies [5]. Some examples of structural violence include institutionalized adultism, ageism, classism, elitism, ethnocentrism, nationalism, speciesism, racism, and sexism [4]. It is very closely linked to social injustice insofar as it

A. Laar, *Balancing the Socio-political and Medico-ethical Dimensions of HIV*, SpringerBriefs in Public Health, https://doi.org/10.1007/978-3-031-09191-9_4

affects people differently in various social structures [6]. To Wadhwa (2012) [7], ineffective/inappropriate policy stances at the incipient stages of the epidemic are tantamount to structural violence.

These must be addressed and overcome for the goals of UHC to be realized. Realizing UHC will contribute to realization of the Sustainable Development Goals (SGDs). For instance, Target 3.8 of SDG-3 is aimed toward *achieving UHC, including financial risk protection, access to quality essential healthcare services and access to safe, effective, quality and affordable essential medicines and vaccines for all*. The achievement of this target is essential to attaining all the health-related targets of other SDGs [8]. Achieving UHC requires key approaches including the primary healthcare approach and life course approach. A primary healthcare approach emphasizes comprehensive integrated primary healthcare (PHC) services which are people-centered and seeks to address the wider determinants of health through multi-sectoral policies [9]. PHC seeks to improve health equity, make healthcare affordable and accessible, and improve overall health status, of not only individual health needs but also the needs of defined populations. Adopting a life course approach has the added advantage of ensuring people's healthcare needs are addressed across all phases of life, guided by principles that promote human rights and gender equality.

The WHO in collaboration with the World Bank has developed a framework to track the progress of UHC via two main indicators: coverage of essential quality health services and the proportion of the population with catastrophic spending on health (defined as large household expenditure on health as a share of household total consumption) [8]. This chapter will focus on one of these essential health services – HIV antiretroviral treatment.

## 4.2    Early Efforts at Ensuring Access to Antiretroviral Therapy (ART) in the Developing World

In September 2000, leaders of 189 countries came together to agree on a set of eight goals with measurable targets and clear deadlines, the Millennium Development Goals (MDGs), to foster global partnership and improve the lives of the world's poorest people. Goal 6 of the MDGs had one of its targets, "To have universal access to HIV/AIDS treatment to all who need it by 2010" [10]. A 2015 United Nations (UN) report assessing the progress of achievement of this goal reported a significant increase in people living with HIV (PLHIV) who were receiving ART globally – 13.6 million in 2014 compared to 800,000 in 2003. Access to ART is believed to have averted 7.6 million deaths from AIDS between 1995 and 2013 [11]. Despite this remarkable improvement, there are significant disparities in access to ART across populations. Only an estimated 36% of the 31.5 million people living with HIV in developing regions were receiving ART in 2013, with sub-Saharan Africa

(SSA) home to 78% of the people living with HIV in developing regions who are not receiving ART [11].

In 2001, the idea for the creation of a Global Fund was proposed by the UN during the first African Summit on HIV/AIDS, Tuberculosis, and Other Infectious Diseases in Abuja. The Fund would be dedicated to the battle against HIV/AIDS and other infectious diseases, with a key priority being to make antiretroviral treatment accessible to all [12]. Since its inauguration, the Global Fund in partnership with others has worked to half AIDS-related deaths and new infections and has provided antiretroviral medications (ARVs) to 20 million people in its focus countries [13]. Due to the expensive nature of ART at the time however, most countries committed to making prevention the primary goal in the HIV/AIDS response with treatment being on the backburner [14]. In 2002, the WHO took an important step of adding ARVs to its list of essential medicines [15] and proposed the 3 by 5 Initiative. This Initiative aimed to have three million people worldwide access ARVs by 2005. This was followed in 2003 by the announcement of the US government to release significant funding – through an initiative titled the US President's Emergency Plan for AIDS Relief (PEPFAR). As of September 2018, PEPFAR had supported life-saving ART for more than 14 0.6 million people, including more than 700,000 children, and helped train nearly 270,000 healthcare workers (HCW) to deliver and improve HIV care and other health services [16].

## 4.3   Cost of Antiretroviral Therapy (ART): A Significant Barrier

At the beginning of the twenty-first century, roll-out and adoption of ART in most countries in SSA were slow due to the high cost of antiretroviral drugs [17]. The issue of high cost of ART is well documented even in developed high-resource settings. A 2015 study in the United States estimated that the discounted lifetime medical cost for an individual who acquires HIV at age 35 years is $326,500, with 60% of the costs attributable to ART [18]. Another study estimated that the total direct expenditure associated with HIV/AIDS care and treatment between 2002 and 2011 was $10.7 billion annually, which is 800–900% higher than expenditures for other chronic conditions [19]. Efforts to combat high prices of ART started as early as 1995 when the Joint United Nations Programme on HIV/AIDS (UNAIDS) initiated a dialogue with the pharmaceutical industry to work toward affordable pricing of ART for poor countries. These efforts later led to the inauguration of the UNAIDS Drug Access Initiative which was launched in 1997 to offer affordable ARTs to PLHIV in Uganda, Cote d'Ivoire, and Chile [14]. The Drug Access Initiative was important to establish the principle of differential pricing for medicines in resource-poor settings. However, due to the high cost of treatment (first-line ART for 1-year cost US$ 7200), very few people were able to receive treatment. Pilot countries employed different approaches to finance treatment costs, ranging from 100%

out-of-pocket payment in Uganda to fully government subsidized in Chile. In a bid to further lower prices, the Accelerating Access Initiative was launched in 2000 which reduced the price of first-line treatment to around $1200 per year. Subsequent negotiations, collaborations, and efforts have further reduced ART costs to less than $200 for some fixed dose combinations in low- and middle-income countries [14]. Key stakeholders in this global effort to reduce ART prices have been civil society groups, people living with HIV/AIDS, governments, non-governmental organizations, multilateral agencies, and health providers. A notable effort to change the landscape of high ART cost was the case of the South African government versus a consortium of 39 pharmaceutical companies in 2002. At the time, it cost the South African government $10,000 per person per year for triple-combination therapy due to pharmaceutical patented prices. The government (arguably) won the case to allow the government to source more affordable generic antiretrovirals from neighboring countries [20].

Currently, there is widespread access to affordable antiretrovirals in resource-poor settings due to generic manufacturers (particularly in India), which have dropped the price of standard triple therapy from US$ 10,000 per patient/year to almost US$ 50 [21]. Also international funding streams which were established to support ART scale-up, notably the Global Fund to Fight AIDS, Tuberculosis and Malaria and the US President's Emergency Plan for AIDS Relief [17] have played pivotal roles in this observed increase in access. Second-line and third-line therapies however remain expensive in most settings. Before discussing the other barriers to access to ART and other life-saving AIDS goods, I highlight, as a case, the journey of HIV-related service delivery in Ghana.

## 4.4  ART and HIV-Related Service Delivery in Ghana

In Ghana, ART for PLHIV was piloted in June 2003. Estimates from the Ghana AIDS Commission (GAC) reports ART coverage of 35% in 2018, which does not indicate any appreciable increase from a 2015 estimate of 34% [22]. The ART coverage for children is even lower at just 20% [23]. These estimates highlight a significant dearth in the number of people living with HIV who have access to ART. Although currently HIV response programs promote the universal access or test and treat policy, only about 60% (113,171/,184,955) of people living with HIV who know their HIV status were estimated by the UNAIDs to be on ART [24]. Ghana adopted the "treat all" policy in its 2016–2020 National HIV/AIDS Strategic Plan in accordance with the 2016 WHO Consolidated guidelines on the use of antiretroviral drugs for treating and preventing HIV infection. This is currently being implemented nationwide. This policy recommends removal of limitations on eligibility to ART, with the hope of achieving universal access to HIV treatment and thus to end the pandemic as a public health threat [25]. The continuum of HIV care encompasses HIV testing services, care and support, ART, adherence monitoring and follow-up, regular supply of medications, adverse event monitoring and drug resistance surveillance, and clinical, immunological, and virologic monitoring [26]. The continuum consists of five main steps: diagnosis, linkage to care, retention in care, adherence to ART, and viral suppression [27]. This concept of continuum of care is essential to assess individual-level care outcomes and ensure that agencies work together to coordinate and link PLHIV to health facilities and communities to ensure efficient service delivery.

In Ghana, HIV-related services are structured along the formal health system – health facilities provide all HIV-related services and referrals along the continuum of care based on the hierarchical structure of the healthcare delivery in Ghana; primary, secondary, and tertiary levels. Provision of the highly active antiretroviral therapy was started in 2003, and the Prevention of Mother to Child Transmission (PMTCT) program in 2002. Antiretroviral therapy in Ghana has traditionally been provided at the health facility level, but ART provision in community settings for those who are stable on treatment is being piloted in some communities [28]. The Government of Ghana endorsed the "differentiated service delivery operations manual" to fast track the achievement of the UNIADS 90–90-90 targets [29]. The 90–90-90 targets were launched in 2014, by UNAIDS and partners, and aimed to diagnose 90% of all HIV-positive persons, provide antiretroviral therapy (ART) for 90% of those diagnosed, and achieve viral suppression for 90% of those treated by 2020. Following its endpoint of 2020, the targets have been revised to 95–95-95 with an endpoint of 2030. Differentiated service delivery in the manual is described as a client-centered approach to address HIV access and service delivery challenges by adapting services to the needs of clients while reducing the burden on the health system. This principle should be applied across the continuum of care to achieve favorable patient outcomes. Recommendations from the manual include extending provider-initiated testing and counselling hours to include overnight and weekend for facilities providing maternity and inpatient care, targeted community-based outreach testing for key populations, and phased roll-out of HIV self-testing. The manual advocates that an integrated pack of medical care for key populations should be adapted to their needs and administered in a non-judgmental manner to ensure comprehensive access.

Some strategies which have been employed to enhance adherence support in the country include fixed-dose combinations and once-daily regimens, case management, and peer counsellors [28]. Owing to the hard-to-reach nature of key populations like MSM and FSW, various public health approaches have been adopted to ensure comprehensive access to HIV continuum of care. In Ghana, such approaches include mobile outreaches, peer educators/community volunteers, and Drop-In Centers (DICs), which provide HIV services including testing, commodities such as condoms and lubricant, information on prevention, and referrals for related services [30].

However, several local studies reveal numerous obstacles to accessing treatment and retention of care in the general population and particularly the key populations [31]. A nationwide survey aimed at documenting the availability and quality of HIV continuum of care reported that HIV testing and counselling services, ART patient counselling, and PMTCT services provision were near universal, while viral load testing was absent on most facilities [32]. The study further observed that around 15% of the surveyed facilities felt that it was the responsibility of the patient to adhere to ART; thus, the facility-level supportive services to PLHIV to ensure treatment adherence was nonexistent. While individual-level motivations for taking ARVs (as expressed by PLHIV) include HIV virus suppression and desire to maintain good health/prolong life, to prevent infection in unborn children, to become good therapeutic citizens (abide by doctors' advice), and to avoid death [33], other supportive services are needed to overcome various access-related barriers. The study by Ankomah et al. (2016) [33] reported that more than six in ten PLHIV encountered barriers hindering access to ART. These were high financial costs associated with accessing and receiving ART, delays associated with receiving care from treatment centers, shortage of drugs and other commodities, stigma, fear of side effects of taking ARVs, job insecurity arising from regular leave of absence to receive ART, and long distance to treatment centers.

Failure to address these challenges potentiates missed opportunities to service uptake. A recent systematic review by Orleans-Walker [34] identified several missed opportunities to eliminating mother-to-child transmission of HIV in Ghana. These included less than expected HIV testing and counselling and suboptimal early infant diagnosis program [35] leading to infants not receiving ARVs. At the health service level, non-adherence to and inadequate understanding of the policy guidelines, non-availability of logistics, staff attitude, inadequate training on the program, inadequate infrastructure, and space were barriers. Clients suffering from various degrees of stigmatization, fear of the unknown, and financial constraints were identified by Orleans-Walker [34] as challenges. Exploring the challenges that health workers face implementing the WHO's PMTCT guidelines, and the experiences of HIV-positive clients receiving these services face, Laar et al. [36] observed that health workers had challenges translating PMTCT guidelines into useful messages for their clients. HIV or ART-related counselling was often prescriptive. Counselors identified inadequate in-service training as a key reason for their outdated and inconsistent messages. HIV-positive clients had confidence in antiretroviral for PMTCT. However, deeply rooted socio-cultural practices and the attitudes of counselors remain as challenges. Related challenges associated with implementation of PMTCT Option B+ in other regions of Ghana [37].

Taken together, these do not augur well for the achievement of the second and third targets of the 90–90-90 or presently the 95–95-95 as outlined earlier: 95% of all people with diagnosed HIV infection will receive sustained antiretroviral therapy. To achieve the third target of the 95–95-95 global agenda – 95% of all people receiving antiretroviral therapy will have viral suppression – PLHIV must be able to complete each step of the HIV care continuum. Viral suppression is achieved more quickly if ART is started within 3 months of diagnosis, emphasizing the key role of early linkage to care [27]. The study by Addo et al. [32] highlighted several provider-related challenges to HIV access and care for clients. Over 60% of service providers reported regular shortage of test reagents and drugs in their facilities, and 57% reported lack of training and support to deliver care. Therefore, efforts to improve access should first recognize these gaps in the current notion of access. These efforts must be accompanied by interventions that address the individual level, as well as structural access barriers. Argued herein, the current global aspirational goal of "treat all"/"test and treat" requires a nuanced understanding of the multiple notions of access and their variegated political economies. While relevant policies exist [36], health professionals providing HIV-related services require training, which addresses, among other things, long-held socio-cultural practices. Thus, health system level, service provider level, as well as service user challenges such as availability of health commodities and resources including health personnel, financial constraints, food insecurity, HIV-related stigma and discrimination, gender bias, access to general sexual and reproductive health services, service satisfaction, and retention in care impact access to services and must be addressed to assure meaningful, sufficient, and sustained access – as outlined below.

## 4.5   Improving Access to Care Will Require Interventions That Address Financial Constraints

As with cost of ART, this notion of access (financial constraints) is relevant especially at the individual level. Several studies in Ghana and SSA have highlighted high financial cost (not necessarily cost of ARVs or direct cost of ART) as a significant barrier to accessing ART [33]. Indeed, in Ghana, while the current direct cost of ART is relatively low, other indirect costs may pose financial constraints to accessing care. A study by Mikkelsen et al., in 2017 [38] looking at the total (direct and indirect) costs of treatment and care for HIV-infected patients at ART clinics in Ghana, reported costs as high as US\$ 112 per patient during the first 6 months after ART initiation which subsequently decreased by about 70% after 4 years on treatment. Out of this, cost of ART drugs comprised almost half (US\$ 52 making up 46%) [38]. Transportation costs are also a known deterrent to accessing care for a significant proportion of PLHIV [33]. Many HIV+ persons are not able to afford these costs. Consequently, patients who are poor and lack resources opt to not access care or do so sporadically which does not augur well for treatment. Putting this in context, Ghana's daily minimum wage as of June 2021 is 12.53 cedis (US\$ 2.07). The number of Ghanaians living on the Ghana Statistical Service report on poverty and inequality shows that about 25% of Ghanaians live on less than GHC 4.8 – translating into about 6.8 million people unable to afford more than a dollar a day. Of note, PLHIV are particularly disadvantaged economically [39].

To address these concerns, some suggestions proposed include scaling up of social and economic safety net programs to capture all PLHIV in need and reimbursement of travel costs for clients traveling long distances to access ART. Targeted social and economic safety net interventions may include conditional cash transfer programs [although there is significant debate on its effectiveness in LMIC [40]] and nutritional supplementation interventions to support poor and vulnerable PLHIV to enable them meet the financial obligations associated with seeking and receiving care. Others have suggested centralization of services within communities or home-based care [41] although this is debatable given that cultural and stigma-related reasons inform choice of healthcare facility [33].

## 4.6   Improving Access to Care Will Require Interventions That Address Malnutrition and Food Insecurity

Research suggests that the HIV/AIDS epidemic and food insecurity (defined as the persistent lack of access of quality food to meet daily needs) interact synergistically in contributing to an excess burden of disease especially in resource-poor settings like SSA [42]. Food insecurity and HIV status form a negative feedback loop, affecting PLHIV at both the individual and household levels in terms of clinical, nutritional, quality-of-life, and economic outcomes. Food insecurity heightens susceptibility to HIV exposure and infection; HIV on the other hand increases vulnerability to food insecurity. HIV also disrupts livelihoods as infected persons often lose the ability to work and generate income [43].

At the individual level, lack of adequate quality food leads to weight loss, which causes a further deterioration in the disease progression and an increase in morbidity and mortality. Weight loss in these patients is linked to a greater risk of death and opportunistic complications [44]. In addition to this, PLHIV may fail to adhere to treatment, due to various reasons, when they are food-insufficient. A study in Rwanda revealed that one of the reasons for lack of adherence in the study participants was a fear of developing too much appetite, while getting better on ART, without enough to eat [45]. A similar study in Kenya on adherence to ART revealed that participants were fearful of taking medication on an empty stomach as they believed this would lead to worse outcomes [46]. Food facilitates the absorption and effectiveness of drugs, and increased appetite is an intended and desirable effect of drug therapy to reverse loss of body mass and enhanced body immunity [45]. At the household level, food-insecure HIV+ persons and their households often have to adopt coping mechanisms, often negative practices, to meet their nutritional needs. Laar et al. in their study on coping strategies of HIV-affected households in Ghana reported up to 61% of households adopting coping strategies such as limiting portion size, reducing number of meals per day, and relying on less expensive foods to manage food insufficiencies in their households [47]. The study concludes that while these strategies may provide short-term relief, they are detrimental, unsustainable, and undermine resilience in the long run. The Government of Ghana through the Ghana AIDS Commission has worked with various partners, including the USAID, CRS, WFP, and DANIDA, among others, to pilot and implement different initiatives to improve food security and improve the nutritional outcomes of PLHIV. However, these efforts are viewed as inadequate by most of the recipients. Laar et al. expand on the gaps in food and nutrition assistance to PLHIV in Ghana: funding gap, coverage gap, and programming gap. To improve food security in this population, food and nutrition assistance must be highly prioritized in this population so that it can receive adequate funding to cover all and not just some of these households. A more holistic and sustainable approach to addressing this problem will be for the government to integrate both nutrition-specific and nutrition-sensitive interventions into HIV programming [48]. Such intervention should aim to address the needs of the entire household as noted by Laar et al.; those other household members may not be infected, but are definitely affected [49].

## 4.7   Improving Access to Care Will Require Interventions That Address HIV-Related Stigma and Discrimination

HIV-related stigma (irrational or negative attitudes, behaviors, and judgments driven by fear) and discrimination (unfair treatment, laws, and policies) are persistent barriers to accessing care and treatment for PLHIV. This stigma and discrimination exist not only in health sector but goes beyond to affect PLHIV in the education, employment, families and communities, and even some humanitarian settings [50]. The UNAIDS has made it a priority to work with governments, civil societies, academia, and multilateral donors and agencies via the Global Partnership for Action to Eliminate All Forms of HIV-Related Stigma and Discrimination, to eliminate stigma and discrimination for PLHIV [50]. As part of its elimination targets, the program seeks to eliminate HIV-related stigma and discrimination in healthcare settings by 2020 and review and reform laws that reinforce stigma and discrimination [51]. It has been argued that the treatment-related 90–90-90 targets, a crucial step in ending the AIDS epidemic by 2030 [28], are not achievable without the prevention-related 90–90-90, which are "reduction in new HIV infections by 90%, reduction in stigma and discrimination by 90%, and reduction in AIDS-related deaths by 90% by 2030". Worryingly, stigma remains one of the major barriers in the development of effective prevention and care programs, to prevention of new infections, and to the provision of care and support for people living with HIV and AIDS in Ghana. Key populations whose behaviors are criminalized, e.g., sex workers (SW), men who have sex with men (MSM), and persons who inject drugs (PWID), suffer stigma both from without and within their subgroups and most significantly from health workers who should be the channels for provision of critical prevention and treatment services. Many people in Ghana still feel that HIV+ persons deserve isolation. In 2014, a Stigma Index Study was conducted in Ghana to provide comprehensive data on the extent of HIV-related stigma and discrimination among PLHIV. The study revealed that stigma and discrimination was more prevalent in the rural areas and that most PLHIV were fearful to disclose their HIV status outside of the health setting in order to avoid stigma and discrimination. The KP subgroup was also found to be more discriminated among PLHIV [52]. The pervasive stigmatization of KPs has been alluded in part to the criminalization of activities of this subgroup (MSM, FSW) [31]. Upholding the human rights of this population and delivering care and treatment in a non-judgmental approach are thus needed as the first steps in addressing stigma and discrimination in PLHIV. At the community level, stigma and discrimination results in isolation of PLHIV which denies them of the psychosocial and sometimes even financial support they need to improve health outcomes [53]. It also prevents them from accessing safety net interventions even when available in the community. In most African rural areas where one's life is closely intertwined with one's community, the repercussions of stigma and discrimination can have a negative impact on life holistically [53]. Stigma also has ongoing effects on the adherence to ART by PLWH, thus affecting their quality of life [54]. Addressing stigma and discrimination will require a participatory approach of stakeholders such as health facility staff, PLHIV, media, donors, NGOs, civil societies, and community stakeholders to design interventions. These interventions will then have a higher probability of addressing the unique needs of PLHIV [55]. Stigma is considered a structural violence that must be addressed. Although less visible, it is by far the most lethal form of violence, through causing excess deaths – deaths that would not occur in more equal societies [5]. To Wadhwa (2012) [7], ineffective/inappropriate policy stances at the incipient stages of the epidemic are tantamount to structural violence. I argue that current policies that fail to meaningfully and sufficiently address HIV-related stigma are equally guilty.

## 4.8    Improving Access to Care Will Require Interventions That Improve Experience at Treatment Centers (Including Service Satisfaction)

The nature (positive or negative) of past interaction with specific healthcare providers has been reported to significantly influence subsequent healthcare-seeking behaviors of service users. This provides an opportunity for better access to ART treatment services for these populations by working with healthcare providers to ensure clients have a positive healthcare experience to ensure treatment retention [30].

Delays associated with receiving care from treatment centers also serve as a major barrier for most patients accessing HIV-related care [33]. These delays are usually in the form of long queues before care is received, resulting from a limited number of trained healthcare personnel and ART centers, select clinic days, and lack of individualized booking system. These long waiting times, sometimes more than 3 hours [56], act as a deterrent for patients to access care. This is particularly concerning for ART clients who are employed in the formal sector and may require permission to absent themselves from work in order to attend ART clinic sessions. Spending long hours at treatment centers instead of workplaces could offer employers reasons to replace such employees and increases the "risk" of their colleagues and employers finding out about their status. There is therefore a need for interventions to address these delays in order to improve access. Some suggestions include increasing the number of caregivers at ART clinics and instituting individualized booking system whereby individual clients can attend clinic at their convenience [41].

Shortage of drugs and other commodities is one of the health facility-related factors frequently cited as a major barrier to effective ART access in developing contexts [57]. Due to shortage of ARVs and other essential consumables, the full benefits of ART may not be realized which affects patient adherence to treatment. This would suggest the need for more resources to be allocated to purchasing and stocking ART clinics with sufficient quantities of essential medicines and commodities. This should also be accompanied by strategies to prevent waste and inefficiencies in the management and use of medicines and essential commodities through such practices as over-prescription and corruption (e.g., stealing or embezzlement of medicines from public ART clinics for personal profit). Indeed, there is an evidence to suggest that countries that have made significant progress in rolling out ART and reducing HIV infection have done so with significant investment of both human and financial resources [33].

# References

1. WHO. Constitution of the World Health Organization. 1946.
2. WHO. Universal declaration of human rights. 1948.
3. WHO. Universal health coverage. 2021. https://www.who.int/health-topics/universal-health-coverage#tab=tab_1. Accessed 14 Nov 2021.
4. Galtung J. Violence, peace, and peace research. J Peace Res. 1969;6:167–91.
5. Lee BX. Causes and cures VII: structural violence. Aggress Violent Behav. 2016;28:109–14.
6. Farmer PE, Nizeye B, Stulac S, Keshavjee S. Structural violence and clinical medicine. PLoS Med. 2006;3:1686–91.
7. Wadhwa V. Structural violence and women's vulnerability to HIV/AIDS in India: understanding through a "grief model" framework. Ann Assoc Am Geogr. 2012;102:1200–8.
8. World Health Organization and the International Bank for Reconstruction and Development/The World Bank. Tracking universal health coverage. 2017 Global monitoring report: executive summary. 2017.
9. WHO. Primary health care now more than ever. 2008.
10. Kennedy P, Kodate N. Millennium development goals|MDG Fund. 2015.
11. United Nations. The millennium development goals report. United Nations; 2015.
12. Release UNP. Secretary-general proposes global fund for fight against HIV/AIDS and other infectious diseases at African leaders summit. Secr Press Release. 2001;
13. Kaasch A. The global fund to fight AIDS, tuberculosis and malaria. In: Shaping global health policy; 2015.
14. Schwartlander B, Grubb I, Perriens J. The 10-year struggle to provide antiretroviral treatment to people with HIV in the developing world. Lancet. 2006;368:541–6.
15. WHO. A commitment to action for expanded access to HIV/AIDS treatment. Int HIV Treat Access Coalit. 2002;December
16. US State Department. PEPFAR 2019 annual report to Congress. 2019.
17. Ford N, Calmy A, Mills EJ. The first decade of antiretroviral therapy in Africa. Glob Health. 2011;7:1–6.
18. Schackman BR, Fleishman JA, Su AE, Berkowitz BK, Moore RD, Walensky RP, et al. The lifetime medical cost savings from preventing HIV in the United States. Med Care. 2015;53:293.

19. Ritchwood TD, Bishu KG, Egede LE. Trends in healthcare expenditure among people living with HIV/AIDS in the United States: evidence from 10 Years of nationally representative data. Int J Equity Health. 2017;16:1–10.
20. Oxfam. South Africa vs. the drug giants: a challenge to affordable medicines. 2001.
21. Waning B, Diedrichsen E, Moon S. A lifeline to treatment: the role of Indian generic manufacturers in supplying antiretroviral medicines to developing countries. J Int AIDS Soc. 2010;13:1–9.
22. Ghana AIDS Commission. 2019 National HIV estimates and projections. 2020.
23. Ghana AIDS Commission. National HIV and AIDS policy. 2019. https://ghanaids.gov.gh/mcadmin/Uploads/nationalHIVandAIDSPolicy.pdf.
24. UNAIDS. Country progress report-Ghana. 2019.
25. WHO. The use of antiretroviral drugs for treating and preventing HIV infection guidelines HIV/AIDS Programme. World Health Prganisation. 2016. http://apps.who.int/iris/bitstream/handle/10665/208825/9789241549684_eng.pdf;jsessionid=96D3C966A85D6B5B4967241613AE280C?sequence=1.
26. UNAIDS. Cities ending the aids epidemic (Issue March). 2016. http://www.iapac.org/uploads/FTCI-Report-HLM2016-060616.pdf.
27. Kay ES, Batey DS, Mugavero MJ. The HIV treatment cascade and care continuum: updates, goals, and recommendations for the future. AIDS Res Ther. 2016;13:1–7.
28. UNAIDS. Country progress report on 90–90-90 –Ghana; 2019. pp. 1–42.
29. Ghana NACP. Differentiated service delivery: an operational manual. 2017.
30. Evaluation U of NC at CHCPCM, Health U of GS of P, Commission GA. A performance evaluation of the National HIV Prevention Program for FSW and MSM in Ghana. 2014. http://www.cpc.unc.edu/measure/publications/tr-14-97.
31. Laar A, DeBruin D. Key populations and human rights in the context of HIV services rendition in Ghana. BMC Int Health Hum Rights. 2017;17:1–10.
32. Addo SA, Abdulai M, Yawson A, Baddoo AN, Zhao J, Workneh N, et al. Availability of HIV services along the continuum of HIV testing, care and treatment in Ghana. BMC Health Serv Res. 2018;18:1–10.
33. Ankomah A, Ganle JK, Lartey MY, Kwara A, Nortey PA, Okyerefo MPK, et al. ART access-related barriers faced by HIV-positive persons linked to care in southern Ghana: a mixed method study. BMC Infect Dis. 2016;16:1–12.
34. Orleans-Walker S. Missed opportunities to eliminating mother to child transmission of HIV in ghana: a systematic review. 2021.
35. Osei D. Early infant diagnosis of HIV in the eastern region of Ghana: stakeholders' knowledge and implementation challenges. 2016.
36. Laar AK, Amankwa B, Asiedu C. Prevention-of-mother-to-child-transmission of HIV Services in sub-Saharan Africa: a qualitative analysis of healthcare providers and clients challenges in Ghana. Int J MCH AIDS. 2014;2:244.
37. Baafi SD. Implementation of pmtct option B+ in the techiman municipality: client satisfaction and service provider challenges. 2017.
38. Mikkelsen E, Hontelez JAC, Nonvignon J, Amon S, Asante FA, Aikins MK, et al. The costs of HIV treatment and care in Ghana. AIDS. 2017;31:2279.
39. Poku RA, Owusu AY, Mullen PD, Markham C, McCurdy SA. Antiretroviral therapy maintenance among HIV-positive women in Ghana: the influence of poverty. AIDS Care. 2020;32:779–84.
40. Fieno J, Leclerc-Madlala S. The promise and limitations of cash transfer programs for HIV prevention. Afr J AIDS Res. 2014;13:153–60.
41. Harries AD, Zachariah R, Lawn SD, Rosen S. Strategies to improve patient retention on antiretroviral therapy in sub-Saharan Africa. Tropical Med Int Health. 2010;15(SUPPL. 1):70–5.
42. Reddi A, Powers MA, Thyssen A. HIV/AIDS and food insecurity: deadly syndemic or an opportunity for healthcare synergism in resource-limited settings of sub-Saharan Africa? AIDS. 2012;26:115–7.

43. Ivers LC, Cullen KA, Freedberg KA, Block S, Coates J, Webb P, et al. HIV/AIDS, undernutrition, and food insecurity. Clin Infect Dis. 2009;49:1096–102.
44. Wheeler DA. Weight loss and disease progression in HIV infection. AIDS Read. 1999;9:347–53.
45. Au JT, Kayitenkore K, Shutes E, Karita E, Peters PJ, Tichacek A, et al. Access to adequate nutrition is a major potential obstacle to antiretroviral adherence among HIV-infected individuals in Rwanda. AIDS. 2006;20:2116–8.
46. Unge C, Johansson A, Zachariah R, Some D, Van Engelgem I, Ekstrom AM. Reasons for unsatisfactory acceptance of antiretroviral treatment in the urban Kibera slum, Kenya. AIDS Care Psychol Soc-Med Asp AIDS/HIV. 2008;20:146–9.
47. Laar A, Manu A, Laar M, El-Adas A, Amenyah R, Atuahene K, et al. Coping strategies of HIV-affected households in Ghana. BMC Pub Health. 2015;15:1–9.
48. Laar A, El-Adas A, Amenyah RN, Atuahene K, Asare E, Tenkorang EY, et al. Food and nutrition assistance to HIV-infected and affected populations in Ghana: a situational analysis and stakeholder views. Afr Geogr Rev. 2015;34:69–82.
49. Ak L, Tandoh A. Not infected but affected: the burden of Aids-induced food insecurity among HIV-affected households in Ghana. In: Rosalie Garner, editor. Food insecurity patterns, preval risk factors. New York: Nova Science Publishers; 2016.
50. UNAIDS. Global partnership for action to eliminate all forms of HIV-related stigma and discrimination. 2018.
51. UNAIDS. Commitments to end aids by 2030 fast-track commitments to end AIDS by 2030. 2016.
52. Ghana AIDS Commission. National HIV and AIDS anti-stigma and discrimination strategy 2016–2020. Ghana AIDS Commission; 2016.
53. Rankin WW, Brennan S, Schell E, Laviwa J, Rankin SH. The stigma of being HIV-positive in Africa. PLoS Med. 2005;2:0702–4.
54. Mbonu NC, van den Borne B, De Vries NK. Stigma of people with HIV/AIDS in Sub-Saharan Africa: a literature review. J Trop Med. 2009;2009
55. Pulerwitz J, Michaelis A, Weiss E, Brown L, Mahendra V. Reducing HIV-related stigma: Lessons learned from horizons research and programs. Pub Health Rep. 2010;125:272–81.
56. Ohene S, Forson E. Care of patients on anti-retroviral therapy in Kumasi Metropolis. Ghana Med J. 2009;43:144.
57. Posse M, Meheus F, Van Asten H, Van Der Ven A, Baltussen R. Barriers to access to antiretroviral treatment in developing countries: a review. Tropical Med Int Health. 2008;13:904–13.

# Chapter 5
# "They Are Criminals": AIDS, the Law, Harm Reduction, and the Socially Excluded

## 5.1 Introduction

Per the Constitution of the World Health Organization (WHO), "…the enjoyment of the highest attainable standard of health is one of the fundamental rights of every human being without distinction of race, religion, political belief, economic or social condition." These words articulated in the Constitution of the WHO, 75 years ago, uphold the human rights of all people to health, to live a life in dignity, and to benefit from scientific and medical advancements without discrimination. Today, gross violations of these rights, among others, mar public health response to the human immunodeficiency virus (HIV) in many countries. Issues of stigma, restrictive laws and policies, human rights abuses, and social injustice continue to hinder access to HIV prevention, diagnosis, and treatment services, especially in population groups at the highest risk of infection, living with or most affected by HIV. Referred to as key populations, and including sex workers (SWs); men who have sex with men (MSM); persons who inject drugs (PWIDs); lesbian, gay, bisexual, transgender, queer and questioning, intersex, asexual, and pansexual (LGBTQIAP) persons; and persons in prisons), these persons are deemed to be at higher risk of acquiring or transmitting HIV. Most of these also fall under the category of population groups at the receiving end of rights-related limitations [1]. Rightly referred to as key populations and rightly so, they are critical to the epidemic's dynamics and integral to its response. However, violations of their rights, social marginalization, and inequitable laws and practices continue to limit their access to health and social services and increase HIV infection vulnerability. Without hesitation, Johan Galtung would characterize such governmental policy responses as structural violence [2]. Defined as violence wherein social structures or social institutions harm people by preventing them from meeting their basic needs, examples of structural violence as proposed by Galtung include institutionalized adultism, ageism, classism, elitism, ethnocentrism, nationalism, speciesism, racism, and sexism. Whereas Paul Farmer would link structural violence to social injustice [3]. It is further argued that ineffective/inappropriate policy stances at the incipient stages of the epidemic are tantamount to structural violence. In 2019, an estimated 62% of new HIV infections worldwide were among key populations and their sexual partners [4]. In sub-Saharan Africa, AIDS remains a leading cause of death among adolescent girls and young women, with very pronounced new HIV infections occurring in adolescent girls aged 15–19 years [4]. The sections of the chapter that follows borrow from an earlier work[1] of the author. This earlier publication of the author aimed to provide an analysis of how enactment and implementation of rights-limiting laws not only limit rights but also amplify risk and vulnerability to HIV in key and general populations [5], which is itself a derivative of a project that assessed the ethics sensitivity of key documents guiding Ghana's response to its HIV epidemic [6].

## 5.2    Human Rights and Key Populations in the HIV Response

HIV and human rights are inextricably linked. Human rights violations contribute to the spread of HIV and amplify its impact. Simultaneously, HIV impedes progress toward the realization of human rights. Many international human rights laws and treaties adopted decades ago include a plethora of norms and principles relevant to HIV and the protection of individuals impacted by the epidemic, including key populations. The international legal frameworks developed since the founding of the United Nations (UN) identify individual rights-holders and their entitlements and corresponding duty-bearers and their obligations. Human rights are protected under international law, regional systems, and national constitutions [7]. For example, the morally binding Universal Declaration of Human Rights (UDHR), adopted by the United Nations General Assembly in 1948, asserts certain basic human rights. The UDHR, founded on the non-derogable right to life, declares in Article 25/1, "everyone has the right to a standard of living adequate for the health and wellbeing of himself…" [8]. Not only have subsequent international human rights instruments built on this, but they have also made human rights law legally binding. The International Covenant on Civil and Political Rights (ICCPR) [9] requires member states to respect and protect civil and political rights in line with the WHO Constitution and the International Covenant on Economic, Social and Cultural Rights (ICESCR) [10]. Article 12 of ICESCR declares that "the States Parties recognize the right of everyone to the enjoyment of the highest attainable standard of physical and mental health."

---

[1] This chapter borrows substantially from a work of the author previously published in Laar, A. and DeBruin, D. (2017). Key populations and human rights in the context of HIV services rendition in Ghana. *BMC International Health and Human Rights*, 17, 20. https://doi.org/10.1186/s12914-017-0129-z, licensed under the terms of the Creative Commons Attribution License (https://creativecommons.org/licenses/by/4.0/).

Based on these principles, a growing number of UN agencies and advocacy organizations have embraced a "human rights-based approach" to health as a method of framing public health policy and facilitating government accountability. A recent comprehensive human rights analysis of HIV-specific legislation in sub-Saharan Africa referred to these standards, noting that the ICCPR and ICESCR's open-ended grounds for prohibiting discrimination based on "other status" can be interpreted to include non-discrimination, based on health and HIV status [11]. Hence, the provisions in these international treaties relating to the rights to liberty, security, equality, health, education, and free and fair trial, among others, are also relevant to the HIV epidemic and for persons affected by HIV including key populations.

## 5.3 Criminalization of HIV and Key Population Groups

In many countries across the world, various rights-restricting policies and criminal laws exist in relation to the activities of key populations. These laws and policies criminalize both their activities and services intended to uphold their positive rights [12]. Most often, antiquated and non-specific legal codes are used to harass, intimidate, or justify the use of force against individuals in key population groups [13]. At the end of 2018, at least 75 countries worldwide had HIV-specific laws or specified HIV as a disease covered by the law, with 29 countries ever applying HIV-specific laws [14]. HIV criminalization has been described as the unjust application of criminal legislation to HIV-positive individuals purely on the basis of their HIV status [15]. In practice, HIV criminalization has a disproportionately negative impact on already marginalized populations, including women. The criminalization of HIV-related events stems from decades of stigma, discrimination, and misunderstanding about scientific evidence on the transmission of the virus [16]. Laws are often applied without regard for prevailing advancements in HIV-related knowledge, including in cases where exposure or transmission has not, or cannot, occur. Sub-Saharan Africa was reported as the region with the most countries that have criminalized HIV, even though the number of reported cases is often low compared to the number of individuals living with HIV in most countries. In the mid-2000s, some nations, primarily in western and central Africa, enacted comprehensive HIV laws. Recognizing the harm these laws do to the battle against HIV, several countries have since decriminalized vertical transmission and confined criminal liability to acts posing a substantial risk of transmission [14]. For example, due to community advocacy, the Democratic Republic of Congo removed its HIV-specific statute entirely in 2018 [14].

Several authors have written about laws criminalizing same-sex sexual conduct, leading to arbitrary arrests and detentions. They note that these laws are used to threaten arrest and punish individuals for engaging in same-sex sexual conduct and sex work [17–20]. Overs and Hawkins once cited a Malawian newspaper decrying the notorious use of vagrancy laws to criminalize sex workers in Malawi. Evidence also exists that in settings where these groups are not directly outlawed, rights-neutral policies result in widespread and discrimination with impunity [21]. An analysis by Persson et al. close to a decade ago uncovered that consensual same-sex sexual activity is illegal in 76 to 86 countries globally [22]. In 2020, 71 countries worldwide were reported to have criminalized consensual, same-sex sexual activity [23]. The Parliament of the Republic of Ghana is currently debating a bill (the Promotion of Proper Human Sexual Rights and Ghanaian Family Values Bill) and popularly referred to as the anti-LGBTQI+ Bill. Ghana might become the 72nd member of this league as early as 2021. Thirty-two of the 54 African countries criminalize same-sex relationships with punishment ranging from imprisonment to death [23]. Viewed as Euro-American decadency, same-sex relationships, according to some scholars, are feared, despised, and regarded with disdain and disgust in specific African communities [24, 25]. Some view such relationships as a condition that ought to be cut out and exposed before the practice spreads like "cancer" among other men. Others have described this argument as the "pathologization" of same-sex relationships. This assertion is evident in countries like Senegal, Malawi, and Uganda that support this [22].

A number of assessments implemented in the West African sub-region show that legal and human rights challenges related to the HIV epidemic are rife among key populations. Sex work is illegal in majority of West African countries with numerous punitive legal approaches, though these are unevenly enforced [20, 26]. Senegal is the sole exception, where prostitution has been permitted and regulated since 1969 [27]. Similarly, MSM are highly stigmatized as same-sex intercourse is criminalized across West Africa and may be punishable by lengthy prison sentences or the death penalty [28, 29]. Nigeria in 2014 enacted a "Same-Sex Marriage (Prohibition) Act 2013" that imposes a 14-year prison sentence for anyone who enters a same-sex union and a 10-year term for "a person or group of persons" who supports the registration, operation, and sustenance of gay clubs, societies, organizations, processions, or meeting [30]. In certain countries, healthcare providers experience governmental pressure to reveal the identities of MSM clients, creating a political atmosphere that discourages MSM clients from seeking care and/or treatment [26].

A related key population policy analysis covering Côte d'Ivoire, Ghana, Togo, Benin, Nigeria, and Burkina Faso (all West African countries) shows that all countries in the analysis except Benin have at least one law that criminalizes behaviors of one or more key populations. In addition, soliciting for sex work is illegal in four countries; sex work itself is only criminalized in Ghana and Nigeria [20]. Non-custodial alternatives to prison are available only in Ghana and Togo. Same-sex sexual behavior is criminalized in Ghana, Togo, and Nigeria, with non-custodial alternatives to prison unavailable in any of these countries. Nigeria has the harshest penalties, while Côte d'Ivoire and Burkina Faso have no laws regarding same-sex sexual behavior. Only three countries (Côte d'Ivoire, Ghana, and Togo) had policies protecting NGOs and service providers from prosecution on charges of aiding and abetting. In the context of HIV, punitive provisions criminalizing the behaviors of key populations not only weaken human rights protections [31] but also limit the efforts of public health personnel to reach these populations with HIV and other health interventions [18].

## 5.4 Key Populations and Criminal Laws in Ghana

One contentious public health and human rights issue that has over the past decade sparked and continues to do passionate national discourse in Ghana is whether or not individuals who engage in legally prohibited behaviors have rights [5]. In Ghanaian society, key populations (as defined within this chapter) face stringent and arguably rights-restricting criminal statutes. Numerous policies/laws in Ghana, including the actions of Act 29 of the 1960 Criminal Code of Ghana and the inactivity of national HIV policies, directly and indirectly obstruct or hinder key populations' access to services – by extension, a curtailment of their right to health [6]. Widespread stigma and discrimination toward PLHIV and key populations have a detrimental effect on the uptake of HIV services, including HIV testing and counselling (HTC), adherence to ART, and access to supportive services [13, 18, 32]. In Ghana, like in other African countries, the dominant opinion of the MSM is that it is a Euro-American perversion that, if not addressed, may taint other minds – noted by Laar and DeBruin [5]. Such framings offer significant obstacles to efforts to deliver services to this population. This mind-set has a large public influence. Local research [32, 33] indicate that important predictors of HIV in Ghana include marginalization, numerous concurrent relationships, stigma, and prejudice.

While Ghana has succeeded in raising widespread knowledge of HIV, substantial obstacles and gaps persist. Among these obstacles is a dearth of data on population groups believed to be critical to the epidemic's dynamics. For example, anecdotal evidence indicates that Ghana's stringent regulations act as a barrier to HIV care provision and receipt by key populations. Such laws are briefly summarized below from the work of Laar and DeBruin [30]. Under the 1960 Ghanaian Criminal Code, same-sex sexual conduct is a criminal offence. Subsection (1) (b) of Sect. 104 of Ghana's Criminal Code criminalizes consensual "unnatural carnal knowledge," where "unnatural carnal knowledge[3]" is interpreted (rightfully or wrongfully) to include same-sex sexual conduct. Section 274 of the Criminal Offences Act 1960 (Act 29) criminalizes the act of prostitution. It states that "any person who knowingly lives wholly or in part on the earnings of prostitution; or is proved to have, for the purposes of gain, exercised control, direction or influence over the movements of a prostitute in such manner as to aid, abet or compel the prostitution with any person or generally, shall be guilty of a misdemeanour." Additionally, Section 275 of the same Act also states that "any person who in any public place persistently solicits or importunes to obtain clients for any prostitute or for any other immoral purpose shall be guilty of a misdemeanour." While drafting this chapter, in October 2021, Ghana's parliament had begun considering a bill [34] that would criminalize homosexuality and make advocating for LGBTQI+ persons a crime. If passed, the new bill would allow for up to 10 years in prison for persons engaging in LGBTQI+ practices and will penalize those defending them as well as penalize the publication of information that could be considered as encouraging homosexuality.

## 5.5    Impacts of Criminalizing HIV on Key and Vulnerable Populations

Laws that criminalize HIV and legal and policy frameworks and practices that fail to protect the rights of people living with HIV, women, girls, and key populations increase risk and act as significant barriers to services for those who need them the most [35]. Criminalizing people for having HIV violates human rights and jeopardizes public health efforts to manage the epidemic. There is no evidence that applying the criminal law to HIV slows its spread. Rather than that, such practices contribute to HIV-related fear and stigma, erode relationships between patients and healthcare professionals, and prevent individuals from seeking HIV testing and treatment. Women are disproportionately affected by HIV criminalization. Because women are frequently the first members of a home to discover their HIV status, they might become targets of blame and violence. Prosecution can act as a deterrent to women leaving violent situations, and some laws are so broad that they criminalize HIV transmission during pregnancy and nursing [36].

Numerous studies demonstrate that criminalization impairs healthcare providers' ability to offer necessary HIV prevention services to key populations and the general population [12, 18, 37]. Already recognized as a bridging population, there is no denying that whatever affects such key populations affects the general population. Several human rights arguments have been made against legal codes that criminalize and penalize key populations and health services targeted at them. In 2001, all UN member states endorsed a commitment to protect human rights in the global fight against HIV and to ensure universal access to HIV prevention, treatment, care, and support [38]. Nevertheless, attempts to advance key populations' health rights (including universal access to HIV prevention services) have been ineffective in compelling nations to keep this pledge. Protecting public safety and morals has long been a common justification for limiting the rights of most at-risk populations. While international law allows for the use of particular measures to safeguard public safety and morality as a justification for restricting certain rights, such governmental acts, according to earlier standards, must protect and promote the population's health as a whole [39]. In the public health context, the legal standards for assessing whether limitations on human rights are valid are addressed in the Siracusa Principles [40]. These principles hold that for a restriction of a human right to be considered legitimate, a government has to address five criteria: (1) the restriction is provided for and carried out in accordance with the law; (2) the restriction is in the interest of a legitimate objective of general interest; (3) the restriction is strictly necessary in a democratic society to achieve the objective; (4) there are no less intrusive and restrictive means available to reach the same objective; and (5) the restriction is based on scientific evidence and not drafted or imposed arbitrarily.

Invoking the aforementioned rights arguments and doctrine, the UN Human Rights Council adopted a resolution in 2009 urging states to repeal laws that are counter-productive to HIV prevention, treatment, and care, including those that violate the rights of population key to the dynamics of the epidemic and those most affected by it. The same year, the UNAIDS Joint Outcome Framework prioritized the repeal of HIV-related legislation, policies, and practices. Additionally, it referred to sex work as a component of a broader human rights agenda [41]. Other world-wide groups have established projects to alleviate the plight of MSM. UNESCO, for example, has backed efforts to urge governments to halt the unacceptable and dev-astating prevalence of lesbian, gay, bisexual, transgender, and intersex bullying around the world [42].

## 5.6   Key Populations and Harm Reduction

Globally, there is broad agreement that harm reduction and human rights mutually reinforcing causes, with one reflecting the other's core principles [43]. The Commentary on ICESCR (General Comment 14, 2000) argues that the right to health encompasses the freedom to seek, receive, and impart information. A harm reduction approach captures policies, programs, and practices that aim to reduce harms associated with an activity without requiring prohibition of the activity, for example, needle exchange programs and condom distribution. Gruskin's work expounds on the conceptual linkages of harm reduction approaches to human rights. Human rights provides normative validation for harm reduction, namely, the legal obligation to act on the evidence of effective interventions to reduce harm and thus protect rights, and harm reduction offers evidence of the effectiveness of human rights-based approaches to health [44]. Further, like others, Erdman believes that international human rights law has evolved to the point where it now imposes obli-gations on governments to provide and refrain from interfering with life-saving goods for their citizenry [45]. A review of the literature on harm reduction and human rights reveals that some ground has been lost and opportunities missed by the failure of some public health professionals to incorporate harm reduction in the discourses of key populations' criminalization.

The neutrality principle of harm reduction calls for a non-judgmental approach to the underlying activity. Harm reduction concerns only the risks and health-related harms of an activity, not whether the activity is normatively right or wrong. In this context, sex work or same-sex relationships are thus not the problem to be solved. Instead, harm reduction programs seek to address the health risks relating to these behaviors (and the negative impacts of a public health systems' failure to meet the health needs of these populations). These impacts include increased risk of HIV infection, debility, disability, and death of key populations as well as the general population.

In HIV programming, key populations are not only "criminals" but are also con-tributors to increased HIV risk in both key populations and the general population. Evidence shows that criminalizing key populations' activities hinders the provision of HIV services to them and is thus self-defeating. Jurgens et al. discuss how crimi-nalization limits the ability of healthcare workers to provide essential HIV preven-tion services [12]. Available data shows that key populations and their sexual partners make up most new HIV infections worldwide in recent years [4]. With these disparities in mind, Persson et al. describe the criminalization of key populations as "adding insult to injury" [22]. There is no disputing that whatever affects key populations directly affects the general population indirectly. In this context, criminalization of their status and actions is medically counter-productive to gains in curbing the menace of the HIV disease [30].

The humanistic principle of harm reduction extends the neutral reservation of judgment beyond the activity to the individuals who engage in it. Regardless of imputed moral status or deviance from legal norms, all individuals should be treated with respect and deserving of concern for their health and lives. Thus, harm reduction approaches embrace humanism, an "acceptance of the simple humanity of the drug user (*or other key population groups*; emphasis in parenthesis is ours), her connection to the rest of us" [45]. The value neutrality of health discourse is explicitly used in support of the humanistic commitment. Whatever objectives underlie laws criminalizing the behaviors of key populations should not require the sacrifice of health or life to achieve them. To do so would be inhumane and degrading. The humanistic commitment of harm reduction applies not only to the entitlement to healthcare but also to how it is provided. Health services, per international human rights law, are required to be "acceptable." This means services are respectful, ensure free and informed decision-making, guarantee confidentiality, and are informed by the needs and perspectives of the individual. Although broadly adopted in criminal legal frameworks (concerned with abstract policy goals of prohibition or legalization), harm reduction is pragmatic. Harm reduction takes a pragmatic stance about risk behaviors. One aspect of this pragmatic orientation is accepting that individuals will engage in the activity regardless of legal prohibition, especially when eradicating the activity is unrealistic, if not impossible. Thus, even if a country criminalizes the behaviors of key population groups, harm reduction practices focus on HIV prevention and treatment. The aim is, therefore, to mitigate the harm associated with the activity. Indeed, the neutrality principle mentioned above and the pragmatic principle of harm reduction are related. By assessing law in pragmatic terms, harm reduction need not engage with the normative commitments underlying prohibition or decriminalization [46]. The pragmatic analysis also focuses on the harms caused by criminalization. Thus, harm reductionists pay heed to the harms that arise out of the legal framework and the consequences of criminalization, such as exclusion from health services, or health and social impact of, for example, imprisonment.

## 5.7    Current Efforts at Availing Health Services to Key Populations and Proposed Future Directions

In keeping with worldwide debates on this issue and building on prevailing human rights discourses and pedagogy, this chapter reiterates two approaches to HIV response for key populations – previously offered by Laar and DeBruin

[30] – abolitionism and instrumentalism. At the very least, both approaches advocate for eliminating obstacles to providing public healthcare to key and vulnerable populations. The abolitionist approach reflects the 2009 UN Human Rights Council call for states to remove and discriminatory laws, policies, and practices that block effective responses to HIV prevention, treatment, and care and advocates for the complete and immediate repeal of all rights-limiting legislation, including sections Criminal Codes that voilates key populations rights to health. The author advocates for this strategy as the best protective of key population's human rights. In keeping with the abolitionist philosophy, initiatives have been undertaken to enact steps to repeal punishing laws, policies, and practices that obstruct effective solutions to the HIV epidemic in many countries. The author endorses this approach as most protective of the human rights of key populations.

An alternative strategy that holds promise to preserve rights – either short or long term – is instrumentalism. Laar and DeBruin [5] articulate the promise of upholding rights (in the short term or long term) through the alternative strategy of instrumentalism. The instrumentalist approach recognizes that legal codes won't be repealed overnight and allows for flexibility for public health services to be delivered to persons engaged in legally outlawed activities, as doing so will ultimately impact positively on the health of the general population.

Outlined below, Ghana's response to HIV, particularly among key populations, may qualify as an instrumentalist approach. Among other interventions is Ghana's "Drop-In Centers" (DICs). The DIC's pilot intervention created stigma-free spaces where key populations (in the case of Ghana FSWs and MSM) could access basic healthcare services, HIV counseling and testing, STI screening and treatment, family planning information, and some contraceptive methods. While a DIC manager with a clinical background was responsible for the provision of healthcare services and the facility's routine administrative tasks, the manager is supported by outreach workers, who were predominantly FSWs. Outreach workers created demand for the center's services and encouraged their peers to attend. The Ghana AIDS Commission indirectly collaborated with various non-state actors to deliver this intervention. An evaluation of Ghana's DIC's pilot project reveals that DICs promote such community engagement, providing safe, convenient spaces for socializing and discussion of issues as well as provision of health services (Bloom et al. 2013). One key factor in the success of DICs as a service delivery model has been the meaningful engagement of the key populations they serve.

Other instrumentalist approaches work to protect or empower key populations in general, which may alleviate the stigma and discrimination that, as shown above, can deter key populations from seeking healthcare. For example, Williamson et al. (2014) present a conceptual framework for an HIV and key population-related discrimination reporting system in Ghana. Aimed at facilitating access to justice in Ghana, a web-based discrimination reporting system links the Commission on Human Rights and Administrative Justice (CHRAJ) to civil society organizations through case reporting, follow-up, and other mechanisms that link people living with HIV and key populations to legal services. In 2016, data from this reporting system show that 21 of 78 reports by PLHIV and key populations to the Commission for Human Rights and Administrative Justice (CHRAJ) were complaints about disclosure of confidential health information compared to three reports of denial of health services [5]. Unfortunately, the CHRAJ report does not provide additional context. To obtain further insights, assessments of human rights issues as well as quality of services for key populations are recommended. Four decades of experience in the worldwide response to HIV demonstrate that human rights-based approaches to HIV prevention, treatment, care, and support, when combined with enabling legal environments to safeguard rights, help reduce people's vulnerability to HIV. A rights-based response to HIV helps ensure that services are accessible to key populations and other impacted groups irrespective of their criminalized status. After all, they are humans, and humans are entitled entities as long as fundamental rights are concerned.

# References

1. UNAIDS: Fast-Track and Human Rights. Advancing human rights in efforts to accelerate the response to HIV. https://www.unaids.org/sites/default/files/media_asset/JC2895_Fast-Track%20and%20human%20rights_Print.pdf. 2017.
2. Galtung J. Violence, peace, and peace research. J Peace Res. 1969;6(3):167–91.
3. Farmer PE, Nizeye B, Stulac S, Keshavjee S. Structural violence and clinical medicine. In: The social medicine reader, vol. II. 3rd ed; 2019. p. 156–69.
4. UNAIDS. Global commitments, local action after 40 years of AIDS, charting a course to end the pandemic. https://www.unaids.org/en/resources/documents/2021/global-commitments-local-actions. 2021.
5. Laar A, DeBruin D. Key populations and human rights in the context of HIV services rendition in Ghana. BMC Int Health Hum Rights. 2017;17:20. https://doi.org/10.1186/s12914-017-0129-z.
6. Laar A. Development of ethically appropriate HIV epidemic response strategy in a resource poor setting: the case of Ghana. Retrieved from the University of Minnesota Digital Conservancy, https://hdl.handle.net/11299/165558. 2014.
7. Boggio A, Zignol M, Jaramillo E, Nunn P, Pinet G, Raviglione M. Limitations on human rights: are they justifiable to reduce the burden of TB in the era of MDR- and XDR-TB? Health Hum Rights. 2008;10(2):121–6.
8. United Nations. Universal declaration of human rights. https://www.un.org/en/about-us/universal-declaration-of-human-rights. 1948.
9. UN General Assembly. International covenant on civil and political rights, Treaty series, vol. 999. United Nations; 1966. p. 171.
10. UN General Assembly. International covenant on economic, social and cultural rights, Treaty series, vol. 993. United Nations; 1966. p. 3.
11. Eba PM. HIV-specific legislation in sub-Saharan Africa: a comprehensive human rights analysis. Afr Hum Rights Law J. 2015;15(2):224–62.
12. Jürgens R, Csete J, Amon JJ, Baral S, Beyrer C. People who use drugs, HIV, and human rights. Lancet. 2010;376(9739):475–85.
13. Amon JJ, Baral SD, Beyrer C, Kass N. Human rights research and ethics review: protecting individuals or protecting the state? PLoS Med. 2012;9(10):e1001325.
14. Cameron S, Bernard EJ. Advancing HIV Justice 3: growing the global movement against HIV criminalisation. Amsterdam: HIV Justice Network; 2019.

15. Bernard EJ, Cameron S. Advancing HIV justice 2: building momentum in global advocacy against HIV criminalisation. Brighton/Amsterdam: HIV Justice Network and GNP+; 2016.
16. McCall B. Scientific evidence against HIV criminalisation. Lancet. 2018;392(10147):543–4.
17. Arimoro AE. The criminalisation of consensual same-sex sexual conduct in Nigeria: a critique. J Hum Rights Soc Work. 2019;4(4):257–66.
18. Poteat T, Diouf D, Drame FM, Ndaw M, Traore C, Dhaliwal M, Beyrer C, Baral S. HIV risk among MSM in Senegal: a qualitative rapid assessment of the impact of enforcing laws that criminalize same sex practices. PLoS One. 2011;6(12):e28760.
19. Williamson RT, Wondergem P, Amenyah RN. Using a reporting system to protect the human rights of people living with HIV and key populations: a conceptual framework. Health Hum Rights. 2014;16(1):148–56.
20. Duvall S, Sanon P, Maeda M, Daniel U. HPP key populations policy analysis: countries along the Abidjan-Lagos Corridor (Côte d'Ivoire, Ghana, Togo, Benin, and Nigeria) and Burkina Faso. Washington, DC: Futures Group, Health Policy Project; 2015.
21. Overs C, Hawkins K. Can rights stop the wrongs? Exploring the connections between framings of sex workers' rights and sexual and reproductive health. BMC Int Health Hum Rights. 2011;11(3):S6.
22. Persson A, Ellard J, Newman C, Holt M, de Wit J. Human rights and universal access for men who have sex with men and people who inject drugs: a qualitative analysis of the 2010 UNGASS narrative country progress reports. Soc Sci Med. (1982) 2011; 73(3):467–474.
23. Mendos LR, Botha K, Lelis RC, Dela Peña EL, Savelev I, Tan D. State-sponsored homophobia 2020: global legislation overview update. Geneva: ILGA World; 2020.
24. Altman D, Aggleton P, Williams M, Kong T, Reddy V, Harrad D, Reis T, Parker R. Men who have sex with men: stigma and discrimination. Lancet. 2012;380(9839):439–45.
25. Sahay S, Reddy KS, Dhayarkar S. Optimizing adherence to antiretroviral therapy. Indian J Med Res. 2011;134(6):835–49.
26. Djomand G, Quaye S, Sullivan PS. HIV epidemic among key populations in west Africa. Curr Opin HIV AIDS. 2014;9(5):506–13.
27. Laurent C, Seck K, Coumba N, Kane T, Samb N, Wade A, Liégeois F, Mboup S, Ndoye I, Delaporte E. Prevalence of HIV and other sexually transmitted infections, and risk behaviours in unregistered sex workers in Dakar, Senegal. AIDS. 2003;17(12):1811–6.
28. Millett GA, Jeffries WLT, Peterson JL, Malebranche DJ, Lane T, Flores SA, Fenton KA, Wilson PA, Steiner R, Heilig CM. Common roots: a contextual review of HIV epidemics in black men who have sex with men across the African diaspora. Lancet. 2012;380(9839):411–23.
29. Beyrer C. Hidden yet happening: the epidemics of sexually transmitted infections and HIV among men who have sex with men in developing countries. Sex Transm Infect. 2008;84(6):410–2.
30. National Assembly of the Federal Republic of Nigeria. Same Sex Marriage (Prohibition) Act, 2013. https://www.ilo.org/dyn/natlex/docs/ELECTRONIC/97399/115559/F-1412838298/NGA97399.pdf. 2014.
31. Global Commission on HIV and the Law. Risks, rights & health. https://hivlawcommission.org/report/. 2012.
32. Bosu WK, Yeboah K, Gurumurthy R, Atuahene K. Modes of transmission in West Africa: analysis of the distribution of new HIV infections in Ghana and recommendations for prevention. Ghana AIDS Commission, UNAIDS; 2009, July.
33. Ghana Statistical Service (GSS), Ghana Health Service (GHS), ICF Macro. Ghana demographic and health survey 2008: key findings. Calverton: GSS, GHS, and ICF Macro; 2009.
34. Parliament of Ghana Draft Bill. Promotion of proper human sexual rights and family values bill, 2021 https://cdn.modernghana.com/files/722202192224-0h830n4ayt-lgbt-bill.pdf. 2021.
35. UNDP. Advancing human rights, equality and inclusive governance to end AIDS. https://www.undp.org/sites/g/files/zskgke326/files/publications/Issue%20_Brief_AIDS-HR_Equality_Inclusive_Governance.pdf. 2017.

36. The Lancet HIV [Editorial]. HIV criminalisation is bad policy based on bad science. Lancet HIV. 2018;5(9):e473.
37. Singh S, Pant SB, Dhakal S, Pokhrel S, Mullany LC. Human rights violations among sexual and gender minorities in Kathmandu, Nepal: a qualitative investigation. BMC Int Health Hum Rights. 2012;12:7–7.
38. UNAIDS, WHO. Declaration of commitment on HIV/AIDS. Geneva, Switzerland. http://www.un.org/ga/aids/coverage/FinalDeclaration-HIVAIDS.html. 2001.
39. World Health Organization. Good practice in legislation and regulations for TB control: an indicator of political will. http://whqlibdoc.who.int/hq/2001/WHO_CDS_TB_2001.290.pdf. 2001.
40. United Nations. The Siracusa principles on the limitation and derogation provisions in the international covenant on civil and political rights. http://www.icj.org/wp-content/uploads/1984/07/Siracusa-principles-ICCPR-legal-submission-1985-eng.pdf. 1985.
41. UNAIDS. Joint action for results, UNAIDS OUTcome Framework 2009–2011. Joint United Nations Programme on HIV/AIDS; Geneva, Switzerland. 2009.
42. UNESCO. Rio statement on homophobic bullying and education for all. Rio de Janeiro, Brazil, Dec 10, 2011. https://www.ilga-europe.org/sites/default/files/unesco_-_homophobic_bullying_march_2012.pdf. 2012.
43. Cohen J, Wolfe D. Harm reduction and human rights: finding common cause. AIDS. 2008;22(Suppl 2):S93–4.
44. Gruskin S, Cottingham J, Hilber AM, Kismodi E, Lincetto O, Roseman MJ. Using human rights to improve maternal and neonatal health: history, connections and a proposed practical approach. Bull World Health Org. 2008;86(8):589–93.
45. Erdman JN. Harm reduction, human rights, and access to information on safer abortion. Int J Gynaecol Obstet. 2012;118(1):83–6.
46. Hathaway AD. Shortcomings of harm reduction: toward a morally invested drug reform strategy. Int J Drug Policy. 2001;12(2):125–37.

# Chapter 6
# Developing Socially and Ethically Responsive National AIDS Policies

## 6.1 Responding to Pandemics

Responding to public health challenges such as AIDS can give rise to social, cultural, political, and ethical tensions. Although such are usual public health challenges, during an extremely difficult circumstance, e.g. a protracted pandemic such as AIDS, these challenges are amplified as public health response guidance and measure traverse the "contain, delay, mitigate" phases of the pandemic. Countermeasures deployed during the "contain phase" usually aim to detect early cases and prevent the PHEIC taking hold in for as long as it is reasonably possible. If the pandemic is precipitated by a condition that is transmissible from human to human, the "contain phase" would aim to reduce further human-to-human transmission by keeping individuals in isolation if they have been confirmed to have the condition or under quarantine if public health professionals suspect that the individual has been exposed or infected. During the "delay phase," efforts aim to slow the spread, and if it does take hold, lower the peak impact. The "mitigation phase" aims to provide the best care possible for people who become ill and support the health system to maintain essential services so as to minimize the overall impact of the pandemic on society, in public services, and on the economy. Each of these phases of a pandemic presents unique logistical and moral conundrums to health systems and professionals. To navigate these ethically, international and national response guidance is needed. These guiding documents or policies shepherd public health actors in the design and deployment of their countermeasures. The analysis presented in this chapter derives principally from the master's thesis† of the author

---

This chapter derives largely from the thesis of the author Laar A. Development of ethically appropriate HIV epidemic response strategy in a resource poor setting: the case of Ghana. 2014. https://conservancy.umn.edu/bitstream/handle/11299/165558/Laar_umn_0130M_14881.pdf?sequence=1&isAllowed=y

© The Author(s), under exclusive license to Springer Nature Switzerland AG 2022
A. Laar, *Balancing the Socio-political and Medico-ethical Dimensions of HIV*,
SpringerBriefs in Public Health, https://doi.org/10.1007/978-3-031-09191-9_6

[1]. Focusing almost exclusively on national-level policies, the thesis in question examined how responsive Ghana's National AIDS policies are to social, cultural, political, and ethical contexts.

## 6.2   General Context

Located on the west coast of Africa, the Republic of Ghana has a population of 30.8 million people, with an annual growth rate of 2.1%. Majority of Ghana's population live in urban areas with relatively higher HIV transmission rates compared to the rural areas. The World Bank has since 2011 classified Ghana as a lower middle-income country (LMIC). In 2020, Ghana's gross domestic product per capita was estimated as $ 2328.53. In 2015, Ghana achieved the Millennium Development Goal (MDG) One target of halving extreme poverty and is "on course" to meet the stunting (in children under 5 years) reduction target of the Sustainable Development Goals (SDGs). Life expectancy at birth is 61 years for males and 64 years for females. Mortality among children under 5 years and women of reproductive age has declined steadily over the last two decades but still remains unacceptably high. A high burden of infectious disease coupled with an emerging epidemic of non-communicable diseases (which includes HIV) is the key driver of mortality.

## 6.3   HIV Context

Ghana is one of the countries in the sub-Saharan region that has made significant progress in curtailing the impact of HIV and AIDS on their population. Nevertheless, the country's ability to further reduce the incidence, prevalence, and risk of HIV and AIDS is hampered by prevailing programmatic and institutional difficulties. HIV remains a significant public health challenge, therefore. Like other sub-Saharan African countries, Ghana has a generalized HIV epidemic, with about 340,000 people living with HIV as of 2019, majority of whom (64.3%) are females [2]. A generalized HIV epidemic is defined as one that is self-sustaining through heterosexual transmission, with HIV prevalence usually exceeding 1% among pregnant women attending antenatal clinics. The country currently has an adult national HIV prevalence of 1.7%. The estimated median number of new HIV infections increased from 19,931 in 2018 to 20,068 in 2019. In 2019, an estimated 13,616 people died of AIDS-related morbidity. Out of this, 11,412 (or 83.8%) were adults, 15 years and above, while 2441 or 17.9% were children between 0 and 14 years. There exist regional variations in the HIV prevalence rates, ranging from a high of 2.7% in the Bono region to 0.24% in the North East region [2]. The Greater Accra Region, the most urbanized and populous region of Ghana, recorded the highest number of people with new infections (5517) in 2019. Overall, urban settings record higher prevalence rates (2.6%) than the rural settings (2.2%). Among antenatal attendees, HIV prevalence declined from 2.9% in 2009 to 1.6% in 2014. Worryingly, there was an increase in HIV prevalence between 2015 and 2018.

## 6.4 Ghana's National Response to HIV

Ghana recorded its first case of HIV in 1986. Approached as a disease rather than a developmental issue, the HIV epidemic initially was managed solely by the Ministry of Health (MOH). Ghana's initial HIV response efforts led to the establishment of a National Advisory Council (NAC) on AIDS in 1985 and the National AIDS/STI Control Programme (NACP) in 1987. NACP became in charge of prevention, management, and coordination of HIV and AIDS activities in Ghana. Thirteen years down the line, the complex nature of the epidemic compelled Ghana to adopt a multi-sectoral approach and a decentralized coordination system for its HIV response. This approach led to the establishment of the Ghana AIDS Commission (GAC) through an act of Parliament in 2000. The GAC is a supra-ministerial body under the President's Office responsible for providing leadership in managing and coordinating the national response to Ghana's HIV and AIDS epidemic. Since its inception, the GAC has developed several National Strategic documents to guide the national response. These include the National Strategic Framework (NSF) I to guide the National Response from 2003 to 2005 and the NSF II, which guided Ghana's response from 2006 to 2010. Between 2010 and 2020, the GAC has developed two National Strategic Plans (NSPs).

Of note, Ghana's response to the HIV challenge has been centered on three thematic areas: prevention, treatment and care, and mitigation of socio-economic effects. There is currently an increased public awareness about HIV as evidenced by findings of the most recent Ghana Demographic and Health Survey (GDHS) [3]. Although the overall disease prevalence is also trending downward, significant challenges and gaps remain. While awareness and general public knowledge about HIV are high, in-depth knowledge about the transmission of HIV is low, and so is positive behavior change. Over the years, data from national surveys show that too many Ghanaians do not know their HIV status [3].

Human rights contraventions, related stigma, and discrimination of persons infected and affected with HIV are persistent [4, 5]. Widespread stigma and discrimination toward PLHIV and key populations reduces the uptake of HIV services including HIV testing and counselling (HTC), adherence to ART, and access to supportive services [6–9]. In response, the GAC's NSPs include guidance on Comprehensive Response to Human Rights-Related Barriers to HIV and TB Services [10]. The author of this chapter and others have previously interrogated of the ethics sensitivity of these national HIV response policies [1, 5] and of the delivery process of HIV services [11].

## 6.5    Ethical Tensions in National HIV Response Policies/ Documents and Programmatic Deficiencies

This and the sections that follow draw from a normative policy analysis conducted by [1]. The said policy analysis identified several ethical deficiencies and tensions in principal guiding documents of Ghana's HIV response. The work reveals that notwithstanding the enviable successes chalked on public health aspects of the epidemic, palpable efforts to address ethical issues remain nascent. First, no efforts are made in the guidelines toward decriminalizing key populations or uplifting their diminished rights. While there is evidence of near universal awareness of HIV, discriminatory laws (Section 276 of the Criminal Code 1960 (Act 29) criminalizes prostitution and soliciting for sex, and homosexuality). The widespread and persistent stigma vented out especially toward some key populations – men who have sex with men (MSM) and sex workers (SWs) are feebly responded to by these guiding documents/policies. There are both political and public acknowledgment of chronic shortage of antiretroviral medications (ARVs), yet there is no provision to sustainably address these shortages or clear guidelines concerning how to ethically allocate/ ration this scarce commodity. Also ethically sound justifications for "geographic prioritization" of public health interventions are not clearly articulated in the documents. Even though all the guiding documents prescribe that HIV services be provided to everyone in need without qualification, the NSP (2010–2015) presented some prioritizations. Using HIV prevalence or geographical locations of key population as indicators, some of regions of Ghana are prioritized or targeted. Laar [1] finds the justifications given for such prioritizations adequate by public health standards but feeble – when viewed with an ethics lens. These issues are further discussed.

## 6.6    Rights of Key Populations to Public Health Services

This section focuses on two of the HIV guiding documents reviewed – the NSP and the national policy. These two documents not only have the mandate but are well placed to provide overall direction and specific protection of the needs of key populations. Yet, specific actions to ensure that these services are key population-friendly or ethically sound are debatable.

The NSP acknowledges key populations as a driver of the HIV epidemic in Ghana. The policy mentions an integrated approach that ensures that key populations access a wide range of HIV services through one service point. There are two-pronged strategies proposed – preventative outreach services based on peer group interventions and curative services implemented by NGOs in partnership with Ghana Health Services.

The NSP and the national policy admit the existence of numerous challenges and gaps regarding how these services can be delivered. A careful reading of the guiding documents reveals the lack of clear guidance and actions for addressing the national social hostility to key populations (particularly MSM and FSW). The NSP and the policy acknowledge that threats of incarceration and stigmatizing behavior toward MARPs by some members of the Ghanaian population are a daily reality. And yet, there is no clear strategy or a roadmap in the guiding documents toward decriminalizing activities of key populations. NSP and national HIV policy have been criticized and characterized as unresponsive [1]. The policies' ethical deficiencies stem from their inactions or failure to provide clear guidance for uplifting the diminished rights of criminalized key populations. Criminalization limits the ability of healthcare workers to provide essential HIV prevention services [5, 9, 12, 13].

In 2001, all UN member states including Ghana endorsed a commitment to protect human rights in the global fight against HIV and to ensure universal access to HIV prevention, treatment, care, and support [14]. Yet efforts at pressing for key populations' rights to health have been ineffective in compelling nation states to fulfill this promise. A popular argument in support of limiting the rights of MARP has been the protection of public safety and morals. The current criminalization policies in Ghana are legal, but they cannot be said to be ethical or non-discriminatory. Ghana is a signatory to all the human rights documents discussed, particularly the commitment pledging to "enact, strengthen or enforce, as appropriate, legislation, regulations and other measures" to eliminate all forms of discriminatory tendencies. The authors of the Ghana's HIV guiding documents should have pressed forward for decriminalization of key populations. This would have been in line with the UN Human Rights Council Resolution of 2009 that urged states to eliminate laws that are counter-productive to HIV prevention and treatment. Even though decriminalization is preferred, a moderate call for unfettered government's support for the delivery of public health services to key populations, without legitimizing their status in the legal codes, may be a start. These issues are addressed in depth in Chap. 5.

## 6.7   Geographic Prioritization of Public Health Services

All of Ghana's HIV policies and strategies prescribe that HIV services be provided without qualification to everyone in need. The NSP, however, presents some prioritizations with respect to rendition of HIV prevention, treatment, and care services. The prioritization is focused on three dimensions: target populations, regions and, thematic areas.

Populations that engage in high-risk sex or are vulnerable to HIV infections based on their occupation, lifestyle, cultural, and gender factors are considered priority for the NSP. The NSP prioritizes FSWs and MSMs for HIV prevention interventions.

Geographic regions are identified as priority regions. For instance, regions that record increases in the rate of HIV prevalence based on local sentinel surveillance data usually qualify. These regions also have a high presence of hotspots for sex workers and MSM and a higher percentage of men and women with multiple partners, as well as those reporting paying for sex. The Northern and Upper West regions were two regions usually with the lowest rates and therefore are not prioritized. HIV prevention is the only thematic area prioritized. The NSP argues that given the low HIV prevalence in Ghana, HIV prevention with the aim of reducing new infections among key populations and other vulnerable populations and virtually eliminating mother-to-child transmission of HIV should be prioritized.

Living in a world with multiplicity of needs, and scarce resources, priority setting becomes a norm rather than the exception. Prioritization is not new in public health. It entails the development of a specialized health intervention approach for a specific group of people, identified by various factors, including geography, race/ethnicity, age, and health issues. Prioritizing allows both health departments and communities to direct resources, time, and energy to those areas or issues that are deemed most critical in terms of need or practical to address [15]. Given this background, readers might want to ask why prioritization as described is a problem. I will like to push readers to consider problematizing the term in the context of ethical tensions that prioritization may produce procedurally or substantively. The potential ethical tensions of the prioritization process are discussed.

The first potential tension relates to process. What is the basis or motivation for prioritization? Who determines what is prioritized? How is prioritizing done? Which of the many prioritization methods available is chosen, and why? A reading of the NSP reveals the first two questions were adequately addressed. The NSP employed both epidemic and situational approaches to synthesize available data and identify the key aspects of the epidemic that the NSP needs to prioritize. The process was also said to be deliberative as a prioritization workshop was organized. This workshop brought together a wide range of stakeholders to ensure consensus and ownership of the priorities identified. Then followed a series of regional consultative workshops where stakeholders at the district and regional levels came together at regional consultative workshops to review the draft strategic plan and provide inputs.

The drafters of the NSP also received significant inputs from thematic working groups, whose constitution was comprehensive and seemingly deliberative or all-inclusive. Membership of the various thematic groups did not include ethicists or bioethicists, probably due to their rarity in the setting. Notably, and as is the norm in the setting, ordinary Ghanaians did not have a voice in the development of the NSP. It is vitally important to include the community when defining prioritization criteria. This question of who gets to make the key decisions in a prioritization process is an important one both ethics-wise and public health sense. In an open democratic society, the development of very important documents such as the NSP ought to follow democratic and deliberative processes.

The second tension with prioritization relates to its unintended consequences. For instance, whole communities or the regions prioritized could be stigmatized just by the mere process of being prioritized, especially in this instance where key populations (who are themselves stigmatized) and high HIV prevalence are inclusion criteria. To discuss this particular ethical tension, I draw on Kass' work. Kass suggests that interventions targeting already vulnerable segments of the population may face certain ethical challenges [16]. Targeting, she notes, may create stigma that some segments of the population or communities or regions in this case are more vulnerable to certain diseases, which might result in social harms, such as psychological distress and discrimination. There is no denying the potential that such targeting initiatives could contribute to HIV prevention, but a possible stigma that it may create is that members of the prioritized regions are high-risk population for HIV infection. This stigma may create anxiety and panic among the targeted population. Viewed from another angle, if a region or subgroup were never targeted with interventions, they may perceive themselves as not at the risk of HIV infection and hence may initiate or continue engaging in risky behaviors.

The alternative view stated above in a way relates to the third ethical tension associated with prioritization, that is, avoiding the sins of under-inclusion or over-inclusion. [17] framework may be consulted once again for guidance. As far as I can tell, efforts to avoid either under- or over-inclusions were not stated in the NSP. Per the recommendations of Gostin and Mann, the current prioritization in the NSP may not be said to be well targeted. The current arrangements affect individuals in the targeted regions who do not require the interventions (NSP is guilty of sins of over-inclusion) and yet fail to include individuals in the regions not targeted who are in dire need of the interventions (guilty of sins of under-inclusion).

The notion of having to prioritize or determine which regions of Ghana require HIV preventative interventions most, and which do not, is an odious one, ethically speaking. Given these ethical tensions, it is only natural that, whenever health programs or resources have to be unequally allocated, they be done with these discussions in mind. The ethical standards and frameworks drawn upon in this discussion if consulted before or during the prioritization process can provide guidance concerning how to maximize beneficence while having unintended consequences minimized.

## 6.8   Guidance on Rationing Limited Prevention, Treatment, Care, and Support Resources and Services

The quintessential and persistent challenge that both public health professionals and bioethicists face has been devising an appropriate approach to ration limited resources ethically [18, 19]. Given that there is universal acknowledgment of the chronic shortage of ARVs in Ghana, the analysis conducted by [1] aimed to find out if there were provisions in the guiding documents to sustainably address the perennial ARV shortages. Confirmation of the existence of clear guidelines on how to ethically allocate this scarce commodity was the second objective.

While acknowledging these points, none of the guiding documents presents a clear, actionable plan to addressing the problem. The national treatment guidelines mention that continuity of supply of ARVs can be ensured by minimizing wastage, leakage, and abuse. Authors of the treatment guidelines are of the view that the current arrangement where Ghana's Ministry of Health is mandated as the sole agency for the importation and distribution of HIV and AIDS drugs and other related commodities will address the problem of commodity shortage. No elaborations are given, and it is not clear to me how these measures ensure sustainability as argued.

The general laxity in putting the needed measures for sustainability may be blamed on developing countries' overreliance on donor support. Like other countries in the sub-region, Ghana for years has relied on donor support particularly the Global Fund and the US President's Emergency Plan for AIDS Relief (PEPFAR) for the care and treatment component of its HIV response. The authors of Ghana's HIV response guidelines are aware that models, which put Ghana at the mercy of continued funding from donors, are antithetical to sustainability. This is particularly critical given the dwindling of support after the attainment of lower middle-income country (LMIC) status by Ghana. National budget statements and economic policy of Ghana mention that Ghana's attainment of LMIC status has led to reduction in very soft and long-term aid inflows and an increased difficulty of attracting concessional financing.

As Ghana's fight against HIV will be a long one, it will become sustainable only if it is owned by Ghana. Perhaps, a report by UNAIDS titled "Efficient and Sustainable HIV Responses: Case Studies on Country Progress" [20] may be consulted for inspiration. The report, which consists of eight case studies written by country experts, highlights countries' progress in making their HIV response more efficient.

The first part of the report examines efficiency gains: countries that have re-allocated resources toward interventions that are cost-effective (referred to in the report as "allocative efficiency") and countries that have made their HIV programs more efficient ("technical efficiency"). The second part highlights countries that have increased domestic resources for the HIV response ("sustainable financing"). Cambodia and Myanmar are profiled to have re-allocated resources toward high-impact interventions in their country-specific contexts. Kenya, Namibia, Malawi, and Kazakhstan, according to the report, have taken active steps for a future with fewer external funds by developing options to increase and sustain funding for the HIV response [20].

To discuss the second theme – who should have access to scarce resources/ ARVs, I draw on the concept, not every HIV-seropositive person who wishes to have ARVs can have them. Medical eligibility criteria have to be met, and so should the adherence criteria. Even for those who manage to meet both criteria, and thus become eligible to enroll into ART, access is not automatic. ARVs are rationed. It is worthy of note here that rationing or prioritization as discussed is not an inherently unethical activity. The question, however, is how it is planned and executed. Given that this is unavoidable in Ghana's context, the relevant question becomes how it should be done. In other words, who shall live, when not all can live? To provide a meaningful response to the above question, I draw on the major ethical principles governing rationing. These range from first-come, first-served to the prioritarian approaches. To lay persons, the fairest way to share scarce resources might be to use the principle of blind justice, which dictates a random allocation or first-come, first-served basis. Experts have noted that this may work only in a theoretically homogeneous context where each person's interest counts equally. In real life, however, this approach does not wisely steward scarce resources. Allocation should be more purposefully cost-effective. Moreover, a first-come, first-served approach favors those with greater access and so perpetuates unfairness [19].

### 6.8.1   Rationing ARVs Based on Utilitarian Principle

The most widely used principle in formulating health policy is the utilitarian principle [21]. The principle's oft-cited statement – "the option with the best balance of beneficial over harmful consequences should be chosen" – according to Macklin and Cowan may be interpreted in one of many ways. Promoting the most efficient way to reach the desired goals – maximizing health benefits of those in need – dictates giving priority to PLHIV whose medical condition is such that they will respond better to ARVs and will be likely to survive for the longest time. This excludes patients whose HIV disease has progressed to a point where only a temporary health benefit can be expected.

The second interpretation regarding who to receive ARVs is valuation of the consequence. Offered by [22] this requires specifying which consequences are to count: is it preventing new opportunistic infections? Is it preventing deaths? Stated above, the central thesis of the principle seemingly simple sometimes involves complex calculus on application. For instance, if rationing is to be done in the simple context of mothers versus children, how effective will, e.g., prioritizing children be overall? In the context of clinical indicators, how many deaths can be averted by prioritizing PLHIV with lower CD4 cell counts (the sickest) versus those with higher CD4 counts albeit not exceeding the 350 cells/ml cutoff point? To Ruth Macklin, a utilitarian approach to rationing ARVs could call for giving ARVs to the greatest number of PLHIV, even if some (the sickest) could benefit only temporarily. That is, give all medically eligible people a chance to be treated, even if that option would not result in the best overall health outcome for the population [21]. The durability of such a process unfortunately is not addressed by the author. It is worthy of note that in settings where shortages are significant, policy-makers and service providers further face the dilemma of relaxing rationing criteria and pacing toward stock-outs or stiffening them to delay total stock-outs.

### 6.8.2   Rationing ARVs Based on Equity or Equal Worth Principles

Equity as a principle deployed in allocating scarce resources requires that resources be shared so that outcomes are distributed as equitably as possible. As a principle, its goal is to reduce disparities in health status among different groups in society

[21]. Such groups may include the "poor" PLHIV, HIV-infected pregnant women, PLHIV from rural or disadvantaged areas, or key population, etc. The difficulty, however, is that allocating ARVs equally among these groups (not an exhaustive list) might not actually produce outcomes that are distributed equitably. For instance, prioritizing pregnant women could save more lives, giving ARVs to HIV-infected key population could reduce HIV infections in the general population, ultimately saving lives and curtailing the spread of HIV in the population.

To expand this a bit, it may be said that such resources should be rationed/distributed not necessary equally among the groups, but justly – giving each HIV-positive person his or her due – in terms of access to ARVs. Analogizing equitable or just distribution of resources with giving each person what he or she deserves does raise other important questions. For instance, how do we determine what people deserve? What criteria and what principles should we use to determine what is due to this or that person? Looking up to the fundamental principle of distributive justice and providing answers to these questions may be helpful in addressing rationing challenges.

The principle of equal worth is stated and interpreted by Brock and Wikler as follows: "Because every life is of equal worth, we must offer the same level of care to every person in need." This thus "calls upon us to value each person's life independently of his or her economic or other value to society or to others, and regardless of social position or stigma" [23]. Sometimes considered a variant of the principle of equity, the principle of equal worth in this context mandates non-discrimination against PLHIV based on perceptions of their social worth.

### 6.8.3   Rationing ARVs Based on Urgent Need Principle

The principle of urgent need is stated by [24] and paraphrased by [22] as follows: "People's medical needs give rise to moral claims to the health care resources necessary to meet those needs, …equally urgent needs give rise to equal moral claims, and…more urgent needs give rise to stronger moral claims." In the context of allocating ARVs for treatment, this principle may be interpreted as follows: Prioritize those who might die soonest from non-receipt of ARVs or those who will be worst off if treatment is delayed. In other words, the sickest PLHIV urgently need ARVs. The moral dilemma, however, arises when this argument is juxtaposed to current rationing criteria where, for example, not too sick pregnant PLHIV are prioritized for full or prophylactic treatment. Although PMTCT, without a doubt, is an urgent public health need, it may seem less urgent because the women and the unborn child are healthy. Of note, the degree of urgency of the need even gets more complicated when other clinical parameters are brought into the equation. While the presence of opportunistic infections such as tuberculosis may be considered in the allocation of ART, patients with acute opportunistic infection on medical terms are not considered immediately for ART. The acute opportunistic infections are treated before initiation of antiretroviral therapy to avoid immune reconstitution inflammatory syndrome (IRIS).

### 6.8.4   Rationing ARVs Based on Prioritarian Principle

The prioritarian principle in the words of [25] requires that resources (ARVs in this context) be provided to the least advantaged members or groups in society. But who are the least advantaged in the context of HIV and AIDS, ask [25]. Is it the sickest? Is it the poorest? Is it the youngest? Is it the oldest? Is it the female or the male? These are questions whose justification – when arrived at deliberatively – will enrich reasoning decisions ethically.

This discussion has not provided an algorithm for use when faced with rationing dilemmas; it does, however, provide recommendations and guidance laying bare the essential concepts for considering when decisions regarding rationing of ARVs have to be made. The question of which moral principle best guides rationing decisions regarding limited life-saving AIDS commodities is relevant and must be addressed. In a morally pluralistic Ghana, it is not unreasonable that reasonable people are unable to agree about which single principle to adopt. Therefore, some experts recommend multi-principle allocation strategies [1, 26] should be considered. However, the most important criterion is that whatever principles are chosen, such should prioritize transparency and fairness. To the extent possible, such processes should involve the public and be made in advance, with clearly communicated rationales.

Taken together, I provide some suggestions that do not lose sight of the various structural determinants of health for consideration – toward addressing the deficiencies and tensions.

First, as a signatory to various human rights documents, particularly the UN Human Rights Council Resolution of 2009 that called for states to "enact, strengthen or enforce, as appropriate, legislation, regulations and other measures toward the full enjoyment of all human rights and fundamental freedoms of vulnerable groups (which includes key populations)," the key players of Ghana's response to HIV should press forward for immediate unfettered government's support for the delivery of public health services to key populations, irrespective of their status in the current legal codes, is reasonable. Scaling up the establishment of Drop-In-Centers (discussed in Chap. 5) will be a key strategy for addressing the curtailment of key populations' positive rights. The policies must recognize and be responsive to social public health philosophy (discussed in Chap. 3). Social public health resonates with today's public health's interest in empowered communities. It recognizes people not only as individuals but also as connected members of groups, networks, and collectives who interact (talk, negotiate, have sex, use drugs, etc.) together. In response to HIV, people and members of communities respond to our programs, in ways that enable them to remain community members – gay, masculine, married, Christian, Muslim, and so on [27].

Second, given the ethical tensions in the prioritization schemes presented in the NSP, I suggest to the powers that be, that, whenever preventative interventions or resources for HIV response have to be prioritized, it be done with regard to the ethical standards and frameworks examined in this chapter. While prioritizations in public health service delivery may not be avoided, acknowledging the potential unintended consequences of the process and deleting contingency measures to address such would be prudent. A development of prioritization criteria (which could include in no particular order priority, equity considerations, burden of disease, cost-effectiveness, public goods, and externalities) is necessary but not sufficient. Seeking public input for integrating social values into the prioritization schemes, and establishing rigorous system for collecting data on the benefits, and harms of a prioritization initiative should not be optional.

While instituting sustainable structures to address the chronic shortages are encouraged, guidance on how to ethically allocate the insufficient ARVs is urgently needed. This chapter reviewed and discussed various allocation principles. These include utilitarian and equity principles, urgent need, prioritarian, rule of rescue, and the equal worth principles. Given Ghana's circumstances, a hybrid of the utilitarian and the urgent need principles may provide the best guidance on allocation of her scarce ARVs. Designated in this chapter as the "utility-urgent principle," it requires service providers playing allocation roles to first be capacitated enough to balance the beneficial over harmful consequences of their allocation actions. That said, whatever principles are chosen, such should prioritize transparency and fairness. To the extent possible, such processes should involve the public and be made in advance, with clearly communicated rationales.

# References

1. Laar A. Development of ethically appropriate HIV epidemic response strategy in a resource poor setting: the case of Ghana. 2014. https://conservancy.umn.edu/bitstream/handle/11299/165558/Laar_umn_0130M_14881.pdf?sequence=1&isAllowed=y
2. GAC: National Estimates. 2019 National HIV Estimates and Projections. 2019. https://www.ghanaids.gov.gh/mcadmin/Uploads/2019%20National%20and%20Sub-National%20Estimates%20and%20Projections%20Dissemination%2021.07.2020.pdf
3. Ghana Statistical Service, Ghana Health Service, ICF International: Ghana Demographic and Health Survey, 2014. Rockville, Maryland, USA; 2015.
4. GTZ & GAC. Stigma and discrimination of people living with HIV in Ghana: a major challenge in the fight against AIDS June 2011. Ghana: Accra; 2011.
5. Laar A, DeBruin D. Key populations and human rights in the context of HIV services rendition in Ghana. BMC Int Health Hum Rights. 2017;17(1):20.
6. Amon JJ, Baral SD, Beyrer C, Kass N. Human rights research and ethics review: protecting individuals or protecting the state? PLOS Med. 2012;9(10):e1001325.
7. Baral S, Trapence G, Motimedi F, Umar E, Iipinge S, Dausab F, Beyrer C. HIV prevalence, risks for HIV infection, and human rights among men who have sex with men (MSM) in Malawi, Namibia, and Botswana. PloS One. 2009;4(3):e4997.

8. Bosu W, Yeboah K, Gurumurthy R, Atuahene K. Modes of HIV transmission in West Africa: analysis of the distribution of new HIV infections in Ghana and recommendations for prevention. Accra, Ghana: Ghana AIDS Commission; 2009.

9. Poteat T, Diouf D, Drame FM, Ndaw M, Traore C, Dhaliwal M, Beyrer C, Baral S. HIV risk among MSM in Senegal: a qualitative rapid assessment of the impact of enforcing laws that criminalize same sex practices. PloS One. 2011;6(12):e28760.

10. GAC. Strategic plan for a comprehensive response to human rights-related barriers to HIV and TB services in Ghana 2020–2024; 2019.

11. Amankwaa I. Are women free to opt out? Implementation fidelity of the 'opt-out' HIV testing for pregnant women in Ghana. Open Access Victoria University of Wellington, Te Herenga Waka; 2021.

12. Jürgens R, Csete J, Amon JJ, Baral S, Beyrer C. People who use drugs, HIV, and human rights. Lancet. 2010;376(9739):475–85.

13. Singh S, Pant SB, Dhakal S, Pokhrel S, Mullany LC. Human rights violations among sexual and gender minorities in Kathmandu, Nepal: a qualitative investigation. BMC Int Health Hum Rights. 2012;12:7.

14. UNAIDS & WHO. UNGASS Declaration of commitment on HIV/AIDS. Geneva, Switzerland. http://www.un.org/ga/aids/coverage/FinalDeclaration-HIVAIDS.html. Geneva, Switzerland; 2001.

15. Rimer BK, Kreuter MW. Advancing tailored health communication: a persuasion and message effects perspective. J Commun. 2006;56(s1):S184–201.

16. Kass NE. An ethics framework for public health. Am J Pub Health. 2001;91(11):1776–82.

17. Gostin L, Mann JM. Towards the development of a human rights impact assessment for the formulation and evaluation of public health policies. Health Hum Rights. 1994;1(1):58–80.

18. Arras JD. Rationing vaccine during an avian influenza pandemic: why it won't be easy. Yale J Biol Med. 2005;78(5):287–300.

19. Laar A, DeBruin D, Ofori-Asenso R, Laar ME, Redman B, Caplan A. Rationing health and social goods during pandemics: guidance for Ghanaian decision makers. Clin Ethics. 2020;16(3):165–70.

20. UNAIDS. UN Joint Programme on HIV/AIDS (UNAIDS), efficient and sustainable HIV responses: case studies on country progress, January 2013. ISBN 978-92-9253-007-5. http://www.refworld.org/docid/50fe8f742.html. Accessed 30 November 2013. Geneva, Switzerland; 2013.

21. Macklin R. Ethics and equity in access to HIV treatment: 3 by 5 initiative. In: Geneva, Switzerland: Joint United Nations Programme on HIV/AIDS. World Health Organization; 2004.

22. Macklin R, Cowan E. Given financial constraints, it would be unethical to divert antiretroviral drugs from treatment to prevention. Health Aff. 2012;31(7):1537–44.

23. Brock DW, Wikler D. Ethical challenges in long-term funding for HIV/AIDS. Health Aff. 2009;28(6):1666–76.

24. Brock DW. Separate spheres and indirect benefits. Cost Eff Resour Alloc. 2003;1(1):4.

25. Brock DW. Priority to the worse off in health care resource prioritization. In: Medicine and social justice. 2nd ed. New York: Oxford University Press; 2002.

26. White DB, Katz MH, Luce JM, Lo B. Who should receive life support during a public health emergency? Using ethical principles to improve allocation decisions. Ann Int Med. 2009;150(2):132–8.

27. Henderson K, Worth H, Aggleton P, Kippax S. Enhancing HIV prevention requires addressing the complex relationship between prevention and treatment. Glob Pub Health. 2009;4(2):117–30.

# Chapter 7
# Making National HIV/AIDS Response Responsive to Social Public Health: Lessons from Ghana

## 7.1 Introduction

Irrespective of geography, public health interventions that seek to address the complex health and social needs of populations affected by HIV (including those infected or affected and their broader network) require collaboration – collaboration among public health teams but also involvement of those outside of the public health system. Lessons from recent global public health responses (whether it be to HIV, Ebola viral disease, or the current COVID-19 pandemic) show that achieving public health goals require multi-stakeholder and multi-actor inputs (including resources and knowledge). Therefore, today's public health professionals should recognize that culturally informed approaches that effectively integrate social aspects of public health into public health practice are more likely to be impactful than interventions grounded in unimodal philosophies. Interventions that meaningfully include community and indigenous knowledge holders ("lay experts") and with meaningful contribution from all relevant actors of the public health system should be on high demand. The publics of public health have unique contributions to make to public health practice. As multimodal models of public health practice continue to evolve and develop, roles need to expand so that all actors are recognized. Throughout this book, I have argued that these cannot be realized if the social is not meaningfully, sufficiently, and truly integrated into public health practice. While supportive of the evolution referred to above, I call for social public health revolution to destabilize the naturalness with which public health approaches (national AIDS responses/interventions in particular) ignore the socio-political and medico-ethical dimensions of public health.

Even for apparently "medical public health challenges" such as infectious disease outbreaks, trying to prevent the transmission of infectious disease involves many variables including populations in their social world. Arguing for a significant intensification of the HIV prevention response, and the relevance of a strong social stance within this response, Henderson et al. [1] address the need to find a balance between "prevention" and "treatment." They argue that effective prevention needs to be firmly located within the everyday realities affecting communities and societies and needs to focus on what is known to work – *noting not just whether interventions work, but for whom and under what circumstances* (emphases in italics are mine). This social view of health has been deemed relevant since the 1970s and has roots going back to the nineteenth century. In Europe Engels [2] and others recognized that disease affected the poor more than the rich and that social conditions were vital in this relationship. In Latin America, the social medicine movement places emphasis on the social basis of health [3]. Aside from being morally pluralistic, Africa is arguably more communitarian than other parts of the world and is or should be amenable to the philosophy of social public health – as discussed in Chap. 1. Communitarianism is the idea that human identities are largely shaped by different kinds of constitutive communities (or social relations) and that this conception of human nature should inform our moral and political judgments as well as policies and institutions [4]. This has implications for our appreciation and application of public health tools to social and structural determinants of health. As discussed in Chap. 3 of this book, the concept of social public health is responsive to both social and structural determinants of health. Henderson et al. note resonates to a large extent, with today's public health's interest in empowered communities. It recognizes people not only as individuals but also as connected members of groups, networks, and collectives who interact (talk, negotiate, have sex – whether it be same sex/homosexuals or homosexually experienced heterosexuals, heterosexuals, use drugs, etc.). In response to HIV, people and members of communities respond to public health interventions, in ways that enable them to remain community members – gay, masculine, married, Christian, Muslim, and so on and so forth.

It is now generally understood that HIV is hastened forward by many social forces. Once in the body, its impact is profound both biologically and socially [5]. Giles-Vernick and Webb [6] concur. They argue that given the multi-scaled challenges that public health professionals face, public health practice of today and in the future must recognize the critical relevance of social public health. And so, nearly a decade following the launch of the Commission on Social Determinants of Health, Giles-Vernick and Webb [6] highlight some of the public health consequences of the chasm between the biomedical and social sciences. They call attention to the need to bridge the divide in order to improve the delivery of public health services.

Herself a trained biomedical scientist, Isabella Quakyi, Emerita Professor of Immunology and Parasitology and Foundation Dean of the School of Public Health, University of Ghana, spent several decades of her professional life advocating that the foundations of public health are solid only when there is an effective use of knowledge and strategies derived from biologic and physical but also social and behavioral sciences. Borrowing from these and other disciplines has led to the great expansion of the scope of today's public health that must continue to embrace all issues that affect social, commercial, legal, and broadly structural determinants of health. Aware of this, the UNAIDS has over the years argued that effective HIV prevention programs require a combination of behavioral, biomedical, and structural interventions. Led by Isabella Quakyi, this revelation motivated the effort to integrate social public health into Ghana's national response to HIV. Described below, this started as the School of Public Health's TALIF HIV Projects and, later, metamorphosed into HIV360 Consortium.

## 7.2   Attempts at Introducing Social Public Health Initiatives into Ghana's National Response

In March 2004, the Government of Ghana, with funding from the World Bank, launched the third component of the Ghana Education Sector Project called the Teaching and Learning Innovation Fund (TALIF). Designed as a medium term instrument of tertiary education policy, TALIF aimed to:

  i. Raise the quality of tertiary-level teaching and learning.
 ii. Sharpen the relevance and skills content of technical education.
iii. Improve the efficiency by which polytechnics, universities, and system supervisory institutions manage their academic programs.
 iv. Tackle the problems of HIV/AIDS by assisting institutions to develop institutional policy and framework for managing HIV/AIDS on the campuses.

It was this fourth objective that inspired Professor Emerita Isabella Quakyi and her team from the University of Ghana to compete for these TALIF grants. They won four of them. This chapter emphasizes one of them – "Establishment of an HIV/AIDS Interactive Training, Education and Development Center" (TALIF Project # CHSR/3/004/2005; Project PI – Isabella Quakyi, and Project Coordinator, Amos Laar, author of this book). Initially conceptualized as the School of Public Health (SPH) TALIF initiative, its overarching objective was to build a capacity in HIV through sensitization, education, research, and information dissemination. The team would set up an Interactive Center, with an IT Resource Library, and a National Toll-free HIV hotline. Together with the other projects, the Consortium aimed to enhance competency and capacities of various stakeholders, increase access to and sustain the use of HIV Testing Services (HTS) in the communities, and prevent mother-to-child transmission (PMTCT) of HIV services in health facilities, partnered with the National AIDS/STI Control Program (NACP) to train HIV lay counselors. These counselors would later assist with the implementation of Ghana's

Know Your HIV Status Campaign (KYC) – offering free testing for HIV to the university community. Following I summarize the various efforts at engaging relevant actors toward integrating social public health approaches into Ghana's national HIV response.

The project engaged with diverse actors of the National HIV Response (e.g., community lay, practitioners, programmers, and policy-makers). Frontline service providers in four Ghanaian cities – Legon, Tema, Atua, and Agomenya – received training on PMTCT, HIV, and infant feeding in the study areas. At the community level, traditional authorities – Chiefs and Queen Mothers – were engaged to share with them, and to learn from them, what it takes to meaningfully respond to a national and a global public health challenge such as HIV. At the University of Ghana, the Consortium conducted Behavioral Surveys to inform local practice and policy. For instance, initially issues relating to HIV/AIDS at the School of Public Health were exposed to a few MPH students who took the HIV Special Elective Course. This limited the number of people who benefited. When the data from the Behavioral Survey revealed low HIV literacy among both staff and students of the School, the project introduced school-wide training to increase HIV literacy as well as the various public health approaches to HIV among community members. Lessons from these activities facilitated the introduction of a graduate-level course, Public Health Approaches to HIV and AIDS. The course explores, among others, the history, epidemiology, biology, and social aspects of HIV and discusses the global or local response to the epidemic. Driving motivations from the outlined initiatives, the course emphasizes the social, medical, and political dimensions of HIV/AIDS.

These initiatives metamorphosed into the HIV360 Consortium – in 2016 – comprising a transdisciplinary team over 50 experts and lay (sociologists, virologists, immunologists, nutritionists, biomedical and social science researchers, clinicians/service providers, PLHIV, bioethicists, policy analysts, community/patient representatives, etc.). This approximates the partnership required for effective evidence-informed response to the HIV and AIDS scourge. HIV360 Consortium continuous to mentor the next generation of public health leaders – equip them with HIV prevention and management competencies (including competencies on social public health). Working closely with relevant HIV response actors, the HIV360 Consortium conducts high-quality practice and policy-relevant research (basic research, clinical research, social, and behavioral research) as well as ethical and policy analysis. The Consortium's research efforts (some of which predate the birth of HIV360 initiation) are detailed in Table 7.1. Such research, practice, scholar activism, and advocacy efforts include dissemination of lessons learned – of both successes and failures. Continued advocacy for a total response is the only way we can close the tap instead of mopping the floor, something we have been doing for four decades.

**Table 7.1**   Select Interdisciplinary Research Projects implemented by members of the SPH TALIF Initiative and the HIV30 Research and Practice Consortium

| |
|---|
| *HIV/**AIDS** Interactive Training, Education, and Development Center Project* |
| *Reduction of HIV Transmission and Severity of Malaria in Mother-To-Child Transmission Project* |
| *Know-Your-HIV Response Study: Mapping of HIV prevention activities to the district level in the Greater Accra region, Ghana* |
| *Performance Evaluation of HIV Prevention Services for the Most At-Risk Populations (MARP) in Ghana* |
| *Scaled-Up Mobile Phone Intervention for HIV Care and Treatment: Protocol for a Facility Randomized Controlled Trial* |
| *Service Providers' Knowledge of Reproductive Rights and Reproductive Options Available to HIV-Positive Ghanaian Women* |
| *Assessing the HIV care cascade in key populations in the Greater Accra Region of Ghana: a pilot study* |
| *Housing and health needs among HIV-positive persons in Agomenya, Ghana* |
| Assessment of non-prescription drugs used among Ghanaian HIV-positive project title persons on antiretroviral therapy (ART) |
| HIV and Commercial Sexual Exploitation of Children in Two Ghanaian Cities |
| Assessment of Diet Quality and Cardiovascular Risk Factors of People Living With HIV/AIDS |
| Challenges and experiences associated with implementing the WHO HIV and infant feeding guidelines in Ghana |
| Experiences of HIV-positive women receiving prevention of mother-to-child transmission services in the Accra Metropolitan Assembly |
| Utilization of HIV testing and counseling services by men in the Bolgatanga Municipality |
| Fertility regulatory practices among HIV-positive women receiving care |
| Nutritional status and feeding practices of children from selected prevention of mother-to-child transmission of HIV sites |
| Long-term adherence to HIV care after delivery among women living with HIV in Ghana's Eastern Region (Nagasaki University Japan) |
| Early Infant Diagnosis of HIV in Eastern of Ghana: stakeholders knowledge and implementation challenges |
| Challenges associated with implementation of PMTCT Option B+ in the Techiman municipality |
| Quality of infant feeding counselling for HIV-positive women in the Ashiedu-Keteke Sub-metro of Accra |
| Uptake of Human Immunodeficiency Virus (HIV) Screening and Antiretroviral Therapy (Art) by Tuberculosis Clients In Adentan and Tema Greater Accra Region of Ghana |
| Assessing implementation outcomes of joint TB/HIV treatment program in the Accra Metropolis: a qualitative study |
| Missed opportunities to ending mother-to-child transmission of HIV in Ghana: a systematic review |

Source: The Author's

# References

1. Henderson K, Worth H, Aggleton P, Kippax S. Enhancing HIV prevention requires addressing the complex relationship between prevention and treatment. Glob Public Health. 2009;4(2):117–30.
2. Engels F. The condition of the working class in England. Oxford University Press; 1993.
3. Allende S. Chile's medical-social reality. Soc Med. 2006;1(3):151–5.
4. Bell D. Communitarianism and its critics. Oxford: Clarendon; 1993.
5. Farmer P. An anthropology of structural violence. Curr Anthropol. 2004;45(3):305–25.
6. Giles-Vernick T, Webb JL Jr. Global health in Africa: historical perspectives on disease control. Athens: Ohio University Press; 2013.

# Index